What in the World is
Anesthetic?

What in the World is
Anesthetic?

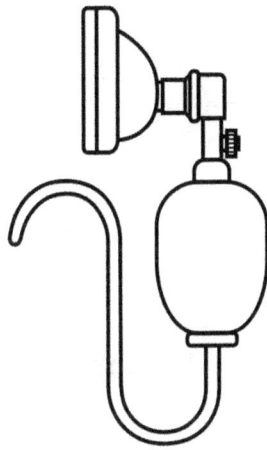

Grace Nzovwa Zulu-Sitima

Timothy C. Chapman

Christina Nguyen

Rico Giovanni Calderon Cuecaco

Chitrini Tandon

Brianna Bedran

Camryn Kabir-Bahk

Yi Yang Fei

Cassandra Van Drunen-LaChanse

Noah Varghese

First Printing: 2021

Typeset and Cover Design by Michelle Wong

ISBN 978-1-77369-231-9

Golden Meteorite Press

103 11919 82 St NW

Edmonton, AB T5B 2W3

www.goldenmeteoritepress.com

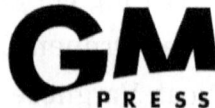

GM PRESS

Table of Contents

Origins from Natural Sources

Timothy C. Chapman

On October 16, 1846, Dr. Morton successfully completed the world's first surgery using anesthesia, administered as a gas to safely immobilize a patient. The word anesthesia was coined by Oliver Holmes in 1846 from the Greek words for "without" and "sensation," referring to the inhibition of sensation that occurs while under anesthetics (Small, 1962). Prior to 1846, the concept of anesthesiology has been explored by various societies dating back to prehistory. Before the development of modern medical technologies, people relied solely on nature as the source for different medical remedies. For centuries plants have been a crucial source of the natural compounds that have anesthetics properties. The Mandrake fruit was first used by the Egyptians 3500 years ago, according to the Ebers Papyrus, it was used for its medical benefits (Pennacchio, 2010). It was not until Hannibal (247-182 BCE), that the Mandrake fruit was used as a sedative during times of war (Stewart, 2009). The ancient Chinese Internist Hua Tuo, wrote about the process of boiling cannabis plants that would then be dried and turned into a powder that was said to disable people for three days at a time; during one particular experiment, Tuo was able to successfully perform a gastronomy while a patient was sedated via one of his mixtures (Salguero, 2009). While Chinese and Indian culture was boiling the cannabis plant, other cultures during the same period, were cultivating poppies in order to extract opium. The opium plant has made a significant impact on world history, with regards to anesthetics, the opium plant has been dated back to the Sumerians who used it as a local anesthetic, and had their goddess Nidaba frequently depicted with poppies growing out of her shoulders (Booth, 1996). With the advancements made in the field of medical technology and anesthesiology, the need for Chinese Cannabis mixtures or Sumarian wine is low, despite this, the roots of anesthetics are in nature.

The first recorded attempts at using natural anesthesia are accredited to herbal remedies in prehistory, dating back to ancient Ethiopia. "In Ethiopia, about 80% of the human population and 90% of livestock is said to be dependent on traditional medicine for primary healthcare services and most of this comes from plants" (Mussema, 2006). The people of Ethiopia, are highly embedded in tradition, relieving heavily on herbal medicine knowledge that had been passed down through many generations. In a study completed in Ethiopia, a group of fifty-five individuals, ten of whom were traditional herbalists, conducted a series of "semi-structured interviews, discussions and guided field walk[s]" to collect meaningful data (Belayneh & Bussa, 2014). This data revealed,

"A total of 83 traditional medicinal plant species against human ailments in 70 genera and 40 Families were recorded. Twelve medicinal plants were marketable in open market places of the nearby towns. Formulations recorded added to 140 remedies for 81 human ailments... About 57.8% of these traditional medicinal plant species belong to ten Families. Asteraceae had the largest number of plant species (10, 12%),

2

followed by Fabaceae (8, 9.6%), Euphorbiaceae (6, 7.2%) and Cucurbitaceae (5, 6%)."

The flowering plant family asteraceae, is grown in tropical and subtropical environments, providing pharmaceutical and insecticidal effects(Okunade, 2002). Fabaceae is a type of legume which aids in secondary metabolic functions, this in turn is useful as a defence compound against herbivores, but also attracts pollinating animals (Wink, 2013). The euphorbiaceae family entails a large variety of plants, from trees to shrubs to herbs, commonly attributed to tropical environments (Webster, 1994). Finally the cucurbitaceae, better known as the gourd family, provide not only a source of food, but the leaves, flowers and roots can also be eaten while oils can be extracted from the seeds (Bates et al., 1990).

Due to the innovations of modern medicines, natural remedies have become less commonly used but not obsolete. Although the prevalence of herbalism contains many factors such as age, gender, ethnicity, education and social class, the use of herbal remedies is more prevalent for people who battle with chronic diseases such as cancer, diabetes, asthma and more (Burstein et al., 1999). "The World Health Organization (WHO), published Quality control methods for medicinal plant materials in 1998 in order to support WHO Member States in establishing quality standards and specifications for herbal materials" (World Health Organization, 2011). Finally, there is debate in the medical community over the long-term effectiveness of herbalistic practices. There is a lack of standards across a global perspective, standards that would determine content authentication, safety and efficacy (Newmaster et al., 2013). Finally it is argued that "there is generally an absence of high-quality scientific research on product composition or effectiveness for anti-disease activity (World Health Organization, 2013).

Since the earliest of times, people have experimented with herbs and plants to find helpful medicinal properties to reduce pain. One of the earliest examples of this is mandragora officinarum or mandrake fruit. This plant belongs to the Solanaceae family, a family which includes poisons such as mandrake and nightshade, to foods such as tobacco and potatoes (Lee, 2006). This perennial herb is native to "the eastern Mediterranean basin and has a short stem and large wrinkled leaves, with clustered bell-shaped flowers and berry-like orange fruit" (Chidiac et al., 2012). Mandrake contains hallucinogenic alkaloids used for digestive and urinary tract conditions, is recognized as slightly narcotic and furthermore has "aphrodisiacal virtue" ascribed by the ancients (Vishal et al., 2013).

The use of mandrake being used as a sedative is not concretely documented, however, it has been depicted since antiquity. Documents from the Ebers Papyrus (1500 BCE), a collection of older sources mentions mandrake in medicinal recipes to treat ailments (Magner, 1992). The image of the mandrake is also inscribed in various tombs in Upper Egypt dating 16th to 14th BCE, as well as depicted on tablets of the 13th BCE where Princess Meritaten offers the plant to her husband King Smenkhkare, who relied on a cane (Ägyptisches Museum und Papyrussammlung). The mandragora is also carved into "a frieze of a priest from the palace of the Assyrian King Sargon II from the eighth century BCE" (Baraka, 1982). These ancient depictions suggest that the mandrake fruit was an important part of ancient medicine, although the exact use of the plant was not attributed to sedation until the time of Hannibal (Stewart, 2009). Hannibal, a Roman military strategist, was said to have used mandrake in war, infusing it in wine for the enemy, who drank it and were overcome by sleep and in turn allowed Hannibal's troops to successfully ambush (Stewart, 2009). Julius Caesar, a century later, used the effects of the mandrake fruit to escape Sicilian pirates (Lee, 2006), while later still, Celsus (c.50 to c.25 BCE) published De Madicina recommended a mixture of mandrake be drunk for toothaches and abscesses(Wynbrandt, 2000).

The mandrake in the time of Hannibal was used for sedation however two centuries later Celsus recommended mandrake for surgeries. It is unclear why this recommendation was made as the plant itself "only has sedative and amnestic properties" but if used in combination with natural sources that offer analgesia, such as opium, a true anesthetic might be produced (Chidiac et al., 2012). Used by many groups of people, the mandrake was commonly used for dental procedures but was also used in early surgery when situations called for cutting and burning (Suppan, 1918). An Arabian scientist Ibn Sina (c. 980 to 1037 CE), identified certain plants with medicinal factors to make a spongia somnifera, described as,

Opium, juice of hyoscyamine, unripened berry of the black-berry, hog beans, lettuce seed, juice of hemlock, poppy, mandragora. Put these all together in a vessel and plunge therein a new sea-sponge, and put that in the sun during the dog-days until all the liquid is consumed. And when there is need, dip it a little in water and apply it to the nostrils of the patient, and he will quickly go to sleep (Haddad, 2003).

In this means, the mandrake concoction could be preserved and used more effectively in surgical procedures. This soporific sponge was seen in various writings for the next eight centuries (Juvin & Desmont, 2000). The use of mandragora decreased significantly with the last scientific mention coming from Dr. John. Snow, who after experimenting on animals and himself, concluded that the mandrake must contain an alkaloid which is the most active anesthetic, better known as scopolamine (Carter, 1996).

Cannabis or hemp is another natural resource that is grown in all parts of the world and has been known since antiquity. The primary source of this plant is used to create useful textiles and rope (Schultes, 1970). In areas of fibre-producing hemp, the plant was not used as a drug, however, due to geographical and climate factors the hemp was able to modify the "pharmacologically active material in the plant" and in some areas lead to the discovery of the resin's drug effects (Information Canada, 1972). This knowledge appears to have stemmed from the Himalayan across through Asia, India, and Africa, where the medicinal effects of cannabis could be explored (Dams, 1996).

In the cultures of India, cannabis was used both medically and nonmedically (Government Central Printing Office, 1894). The use of cannabis was more prevalent during the festival of Durga Puja, but occasions such as marriages and births were also appropriate to use cannabis to "induce a relaxed and sociable mood, and a good appetite" (Kalant, 2001). It was more customary to use weaker preparations such as ëbhangí (comparable to marijuana) was taken by mouth, and the slightly stronger preparation ëganjaí was smoked (Kalant, 2001). The most potent preparation, ëcharasí (known elsewhere as hashish) was not used for these purposes as it was only used by the social outcasts(Kalant, 2001). It is also notable that cannabis was a part of the therapeutic armamentarium in traditional Indian medicine, being used as a sedative, relaxant, appetite stimulant, aiding in opiate withdrawal among other remedies (Kalant, 1972).

Comparably in China, during the same time, hemp was used mostly for its fibre, but was permitted in Taoist ritual incense burners. It is suggested that the "ancient Teoists experimented systematically with hallucinogenic smokes" (Needham, 1974). It is rumored that Lady Wei Huacun and Xu Mi, who founded the Taoist Shangqing School received scriptural revelations from immortals while "aided most certainly by cannabis" (Needham, 1974). In most cases of the Taoist uses of cannabis, the plant flowers were consumed to induce hallucination experiences (Needham et al., 1980).

Cannabis is still used in modern societies, however, it has become more popular in both social and medicinal contexts. It is becoming increasingly more common for cannabis to be a decriminalized or legal substance, which has further increased the variety of uses and users (Fritz, 2021). With a wide variety of pharmacological effects, cannabis can be used to treat a wide variety of chronic illnesses. One such chronic illness included glaucoma, where a study showed that 65 percent of normal and glaucoma affected participants were able to see decreased intraocular pressure (IOP) from both oral THC and smoking marigiuana (Green, 1998). With increased legalization further restrictions are able to be put in place from production to marketing which makes it more trustworthy at the consumer level (Health Canada, 2016).

Opium is among the oldest natural sources of anesthetics in the world, with recorded use of opium being found in Europe, Africa and Asia. Opium is sourced from the poppy plant which is known to grow in the Middle East, India, Europe, and China among other places around the world. The Poppy plant is grown until the pods are large enough to be scored two-three times in order to drain the milky latex substance that is then dried, this dried latex is opium and can then be chemically processed into other substances such as heroin. Opium is popular as a local anesthetic due to its high percentage of analgesic alkaloid morphine, codeine and thebaine which act as painkillers when ingested in the right amount.

The first cultivation of poppies was done by the Summarians who would drain the poppies in the morning, allow the latex to dry during the afternoon, making opium by the evening; the Summarians called the poppy plant "hul gil" or the "joy plant" (Brownstein, 1993). Following along with the Summarians, the Assyrians, Babylonians, and Egyptians all cultivated poppies

7

in order to mass produce opium. Opium was used in religious ceremonies as a way to prove the healing powers of the religious leaders, as well as a medical treatment for several illnesses. The Egyptians used opium as an economic resource, with records stating that the Phoenicians and Minoans traded around the Mediterranean Sea, including to Greece, Carthage, and Europe (Kritikos & Papadaki, 1967).

With the Egyptians introducing opium to the trading market, opium reached the lands south and east of the Medditarian Sea, where the Islamic Societies became very familiar with the poppy plant. According to Dioscorides' five-volume De Materia Medica, opium had a wide range of medical uses by the Islamic people, from a general pain revealer to a sleep aid. The Arabic physician Muhammad Ibn Zakariya al-Razi (845-930 AD) was a student of Galel and believed that Opium could be used as an at-home treatment for melancholy in the absence of a doctor. Al-Razi was able to author an at home medical manual which was written for the ordinary citizen for self-admission if a physician was not able to assist (A Jewish Virtual Library, 2008). Another Arabic physician described opium as the most powerful of the estupefacientes, in comparison to the Mandrake fruit and other highly effective herbs (Heydari et al., 2013).

Since its usage as an ancient pain reliever and in religious ceremonies, opium derived from poppies has been the cause of several conflicts but also has been the source of various positive medical advances. In 1804 Friedrich Wilhelm Adam Sertürner was the first to isolate morphine from the opium poppy and within fifty years the use of opium as a sedative was slowing, due to the introduction of purified synthetic opiates (Morimoto et al., 2001). Despite the production and surreal effectiveness of synthetic opiates, straight morphine is the preferred drug of choice by combat medics, as morphine has unmatched pain-relieving properties (Operational Medicine, 1999).

The curiosity surrounding the natural sources of anesthetics has been seen in all major societies throughout history. The first official use of anesthetics being used in surgeries was in the 1840's by dentists. Before people relied on medical technology, anesthetics were sourced naturally, the Summarians used opium as both a source of pain relief as well as in religious ceremonies. Cannabis was used by the ancient Indians and Chinese as a mixture for ceremonial use in order to stimulate appetites and reach a new level of relaxation. The Egyptians and Romans used the Mandrake fruit as a sedative, with Hannibal being the first to use it as an anesthetic in battle. The advancement made in the field of medicine throughout the last two hundred years have steered society away from the natural sources of anesthetics, but it is critical to remember how and where it all began.

The Discovery of Diethyl Ether as an Anaesthetic

Christina Nguyen

This chapter will place the discovery of diethyl ether as an anaesthetic within the wider context of anesthesiology. This means that the discussion will first focus on context, then the discovery, then the uses, and the benefits and challenges of using diethyl ether. These usages of the anesthetic include both in the developed and developing world, in relation to economic feasibility.

Historical Context of Anaesthesia

Discoveries

Before 1846, in the West, there were few known ways to provide anaesthesia to those undergoing surgery (Watson & Stetka, 2016). General references to pain-relieving methods in surgery involved healing-women's plants and herbs, rather than rigorous scientific discovery of medicines. The process of surgery was extraordinarily painful, bloody, and unhygienic (especially as the theory of germs and immunology was not fully developed, and the miasma theory was widely preferred) (Minkowski, 1992). Surgeons were praised for their speed, rather than skill or successful completion of operation. The Massachusetts General Hospital (MGH) was the busiest surgical center in North America. It is there that we see the breakthroughs in anaesthesia occurring.

The father of anaesthesiology is considered to be Horace Wells, who, in 1844, was a dentist. He attended a party, where he observed that party-goers who inhaled nitrous oxide (N2O) would not suffer pain when injured. He then went on to use nitrous oxide in his dental practice, and had his own tooth extracted under nitrous oxide anaesthesia. In 1845, he proposed nitrous oxide as a possible anaestheisa to the committee at MGH. Sadly, it was an abysmal failure, as nitrous oxide was not a strong enough anaesthesia (Haridas, 2013). Dr. William Morton, at the same time as Wells, was also a dentist. He successfully demonstrated a tumor removal under ether anaesthesia in 1845. Morton's name was made from this success. So that started general aneasthesia for general surgery, using ether (today the specific compound is diethyl ether) (The Editors of Encyclopaedia Britannica, 1998). This can be observed in Figure 1.

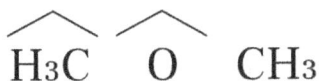

$$H_3C \quad O \quad CH_3$$

figure 1. Diethyl ether's chemical makeup.

The other area laid aside in all of this was obstetrical anaesthesia. Partly this was due to the religious bias in which women were expected to bear pain during birth as recompense for original sin (King James Version, Gen. 3:16). However, England's Queen Victoria was famously not in favor of giving birth in pain, and so she gave birth to her eighth child, Princess Beatrice, under the influence of chloroform in 1853 under Dr. John Snow (Frercihs, n.d.). From that moment forward, obstetrical anaesthesia had a solid place in medicine.

Today, however, diethyl ether is rarely used – for several excellent reasons we will discuss later in this paper.

Uses
Originally, the mask and gauze worked to give patients ether in a style known as the Schimmelbusch mask, named after the German physician who initially developed it (Wood Library Museum, n.d.). It was an open breathing system into which the anesthesia could be dropped slowly. The patient would breathe the vapor. Today the anesthetic system is more complex, with many devices that provide warning signs in case the patient should be affected negatively by the administration of anesthesia.

Discovery of Diethyl Ether

Ether, known alternatively as diethyl ether, was first recorded to have been prepared by Valerius Cordus, a botanist, in the mid-1500s. At the time, it was called sulfuric ether, because it was made from the distillation of the oil of vitriol (which contained sulfur) and a wine. It became a recreational drug in Britain's lower classes, as a replacement for alcohol (Encyclopedia.com, 2016). This method moved overseas and Americans, in the 1800s, would use ether as a way to lose consciousness by holding soaked towels to their faces.

In 1842, we have records of diethyl ether being used as a general anesthetic by Dr. Crawford Williamson Long. He removed a tumor from a patient's neck, but his papers were not published until long after, so he is sometimes forgotten as being the first.

As previously mentioned, the first proper demonstration of ether as an inhalation (that is, breathing in, rather than an injected anesthetic) anesthetic was in October of 1846 by

William Morton, the Bostonian dentist, followed rapidly by Dr. Wells.

The Uses of Diethyl Ether

In the developed world

In the Western world, diethyl ether is no longer taught to be a general anaesthetic. There are many high-risk factors in its use that renders it simply unfavorable for use. First, it often irritates mucous membranes (e.g. throat, nose of patients) and cause violent coughing and hypersalivation (excessive drooling). Secondly, and more importantly, it is very flammable; in modern surgical rooms, there are many electronics that increase the risk of fires. In some cases, it raises pressure intercranial (inside the brain), causing convulsions and potential permanent damage (Science Direct, 1920).

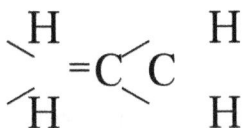

figure 2. ethylene

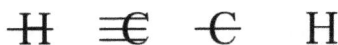

figure 3. acetylene

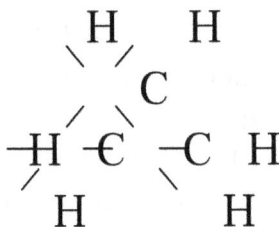

figure 4. cyclopropane

Furthermore, its flammability also means that it causes violent explosions, which are certainly not helpful to the operating room. Much has been recorded about such unfortunate experiences. Indeed, in 1850 we have a recorded fire that happened as a result of anaesthetic use, when ether caught fire (McGill, n.d.). After this, a whole rash of fires and explosions were recorded, due to various flammable types of anaesthetic (and not just diethyl ether). This included ethylene (C_2H_4), acetylene (C_2H_2), and cyclopropane (C_3H_6). Taking a look at the chemical structures of all these anesthetics in Figures 2 – 4, we can see that they are flammable because of the carbon and hydrogen, which recombines easily with oxygen (which is required for fires to start).

Though some early incidents were frightening rather than causing serious injuring, the following cases with death helped urge along the decision to stop the use of flammable anesthetics, including diethyl ether, in the operating room. Now the use of these chemicals are very infrequent, and used in exceptional cases, such as in developing countries, where there are few suitable alternatives. The following section will therefore discuss some of these cases.

In developing and underdeveloped nations
Humanitarian crises included, shortages of people trained in anaesthetics poses a large risk to operations carried out in developing and underdeveloped nations. Largely this stems from a lack of priority for anaesthesia, in favor of the traditional image of a doctor who provides healthcare in a general manner. Indeed, surgical operating rooms are widely considered inadequate when compared to American standards (O. Akenroye, Adebona, & Akenroye, 2013). Basic medical equipment, even just for observing vital signs, are woefully undersupplied.

Furthermore, since anesthesiologists are in short supply in third-world countries, anaesthesia is often administered by nurses under the supervision of a surgeon. With little formal training in anesthesiology, this increases risks incurred by the patient. Developing countries have had to make cost-cutting cuts in order to provide anaesthesia. Endotracheal tubes, for example, are reused and recycled several times before becoming harmful due to balloon rupture after a few uses (al., 2009).

The mainstay of western anesthesiology, expensive anaesthetic vaporizers, have been largely abandoned. These devices are costly to purchase and maintain. Over time, many parts will have to be replaced consistently to ensure a standard level of operation. This is, for obvious financial reasons, typically unreasonable for developing and underdeveloped nations. Furthermore, these vaporizers need a constant supply of oxygen, which is not always available in developing countries, as we have already observed in India with the current COVID-19 crisis (Bhandari, et al., 2020). As a result, draw-over anaesthesia is frequently used. The carrier gas (atmospheric, or just plain room air) is drawn over the volatile liquid (anaesthetic chemical) by the patients' respiratory efforts in draw-over anaesthesia. Drawover systems are easy to set up and operate. The drawover technique is, above all, safe for patients.

Anesthetic medications, which are popular in western anesthesiology, are scarce in developing countries. The fluorinated hydrocarbons sevoflurane, desflurane, and isoflurane, which are the main inhalation agents in the West, are not available in developing countries. These agents are both costly and need a lot of equipment to distribute them. Rather, halothane is the most commonly used volatile agent in developing nations.

These agents are both costly and need a lot of equipment to distribute them. Instead, in developed countries, halothane is the most commonly used volatile agent. Ether is also used, but its use is restricted due to its scarcity and flammability. Substituting ether for halothane in developing countries, especially in those that already use drawover anaesthesia, may save money while also improving surgical anaesthesia safety.

In humanitarian settings
The author would like to point out that little has been done to research the uses of particular types of anaesthesia, let alone diethyl ether, in humanitarian settings, such as with Médicins sans Frontiers. There is little doubt that regional, political, and cultural challenges arise in the procurement and use of anesthetics in humanitarian settings, possibly also because it is not always considered essential nor a priority for supplies. What the author has found, however, is that much research has been done on how underprepared and undersupplied anesthesiologists feel when working in such areas (Rössler, Marhofer, Hüpfl, Peterhans, & Schebesta, 2013).

Benefits and Challenges of Using Diethyl Ether

Ether versus halothane
Although abandoned in western anesthesia, ether has long been known as a relatively safe and inexpensive anesthetic. Halothane costs approximately U.S. $140 per liter (U.S. $0.14 per ml). Ether comes at a cost of about $2.24 USD per hour of use. This is a considerable portion of the small budget of anesthesiology departments in developing nations. Ether, on the other hand, is just $10 per liter. Using the same figures as before, this will cost US $0.16 per hour of usage (an increase of US $2.08 per hour over halothane). Thousands of dollars a year could be saved by struggling anesthesiology departments as a result of the cost gap (Beringer, 2008).

By using diethyl ether as an anaesthetic instead of the costly, first-world alternatives, hospitals in rural areas could save money as well, and save more patients with the same small budget. Although halothane is relatively costly to produce and must be processed in large factories before being shipped to rural health care facilities, ether can be easily and inexpensively produced locally from ethanol. Buying locally produced anaesthetic ether could have a huge impact on costs, local economies, and the self-sufficiency of rural hospitals in developing countries.

Using drawover anaesthetic procedures, both halothane and ether can be conveniently administered. However, without intra-operative control, halothane is a relatively dangerous agent to use. As previously mentioned, developing countries seldom have a sufficient supply of oxygen or electricity. Ether is a sympathomimetic agonist, meaning it increases cardiac activity, respiratory rate, and bronchodilation. When supplemental oxygen, endotracheal intubation, and cardiac monitoring are not available, ether is a safe alternative.

Finally, as opposed to halothane, the side effects of ether anaesthesia are relatively minor. Halothane hepatitis is a well-known side effect in patients who have been exposed to the drug. While halothane hepatitis is relatively uncommon (affecting just 1/10,000 patients), it has a 50% mortality rate. Furthermore, halothane has been linked to cardiac arrhythmias and fatal bradycardia. Halothane has been largely phased out of adult use in the United States and many other countries due to concerns about its hepatotoxicity. Newer, safer volatile anaesthetics gradually supplanted halothane. However, due to its low cost, halothane continues to play an important role in countries with varying medical and legal climates. In Iran, for example, halothane is still used as the primary anaesthetic in more than 80% of hospitals. As a result, halothane hepatitis is becoming more prevalent in Iran and other countries that still use the gas. Ether, on the other hand, is a relatively safe drug, with the most common side effects being nausea and vomiting after the surgery is performed.

This occurs in the majority of patients who were exposed to diethyl ether.

To tackle the ether's flammability, operating rooms in developing countries can mandate some reasonably simple precautions. Open flames, such as those generated by alcohol lamps, Bunsen burners, matches, and smoking, must be avoided in rooms where anaesthetics are administered or present. Plus, to prevent fires caused by sunlight's heating properties, ether should be contained in dark bottles, preferably made of glass.

Obstacles to global adoption of diethyl ether as an anaesthetic

Though halothane is now the most commonly used volatile agent in developed countries, ether is still used in others. Unfortunately, due to a lack of ether availability and medical provider education in ether anaesthesia, even this usage is jeopardised. Many aspiring anesthesiologists have been turned away due to a lack of support for anaesthesia departments in developing countries.

Unfortunately, ether anaesthesia and drawover procedures are no longer taught in first-world countries' curricula. This leads to medical migration; anesthesiologists trained in developed countries frequently stay in the countries where they were trained after completing their education. Furthermore, like in most fields of humanitarian aid, volunteer practitioners from the West who travel to developing countries are unfamiliar with ether and drawover techniques and are often unprepared to cope with the realities of anaesthesia delivery in the developing world. In recent years, anaesthetic ether has also become scarce. Due to dwindling demand for the low-cost agent in developing countries, several manufacturers have decided to discontinue production.

For Further Consideration

The reader may wish to look into these areas for further information on the history of anaesthesia and ether's use in medicine: use of anesthetics of humanitarian crises, and use of ether in military campaigns during the nineteenth and twentieth centuries.

Everyday Use in Surgeries

Rico Giovanni Calderon Cuecaco

The everyday use of anesthetics for surgeries is one of the major signs of progress in modern medicine. On October 16, 1846, Dr. Morton and John Collins Warren completed the first surgical procedure with anesthesia. Dr. Morton single-handedly proved that effective use of gas with the proper dose can temporarily immobilize patients to provide a safe and successful approach to surgical procedures. The historical discovery and use of anesthetics changed the medical landscape and approaches to new surgical procedures, thereby allowing doctors to complete rigorous surgeries with the use of anesthesia. The surgical innovation of anesthetics evoked controversy and generated discussions regarding the safety and side effects of patients who underwent surgery with anesthesia. Many believe that Anesthetics is somewhat a form of a narcotic which causes the patient to become "zombified" and left in a state of vulnerability. According to Wikipedia, anesthesia is Greek for "without sensation". It is a state of controlled, temporary loss of sensation or awareness induced for medical purposes. It may include some or all analgesia (relief from or prevention of pain), paralysis (muscle relaxation), amnesia (loss of memory), and unconsciousness. Anesthetics alone changed the ways of understanding within the medical field as doctors, surgeons, and scholarly medical professionals through the idea of intentional immobilization of patients. Throughout this chapter, areas surrounding the everyday use of anesthetics in surgeries will be explored by explaining and understanding general anesthetics, the pros & cons, how and why did anesthesia came to be, and why is anesthesia the primary approach to everyday surgical procedures.

What is General Anesthetics?

General anesthetics can be defined as an artificial substance induced by the administration of gases or the injection of drugs before surgical operations. This allows the patient to become insensitive to pain before the surgery and allows the patient to become less receptive to the pain of post-surgery. According to Dr. Damien Jones Wilson, "anesthesia makes an area of the body numb to prevent the patient from feeling pain." (Wilson, 2018). The administration of anesthetics can completely block sensation to the area of the body that requires surgery. The anesthesiologist injects local anesthesia near the cluster of nerves that provides sensations to that area. The use of anesthesia has allowed surgeons to work on patients without the unfortunate event of the patient waking up mid-procedure. Before the innovative incorporation of anesthetics, the first attempts of medically induced immobilization consisted of herbal remedies administered through smoke or digested. Alcohol is also one of the oldest known sedatives that surgeons used in surgical procedures. In some cases, patients during this time in history would find themselves awake mid-procedure while the surgeon is cutting the inside of their body. The modern use of anesthesia helps patients undergo surgical procedures in a deep, medically induced slumber, preventing the brain from processing pain and from remembering what happened during the surgery. While there are many types and levels of anesthesia — medication to keep you from feeling pain during surgery — general anesthesia is most commonly used during major operations, such as knee and hip replacements, heart surgeries and many types of surgical procedures to treat cancer. (Wilson, 2018) Although anesthesia is beneficial for patients and surgeons, there is also a slim chance that patients could wake up during the procedure. Despite the historical use of early anesthetics and a few recorded cases where patients felt the pain while undergoing surgical procedures, patients under modern anesthetics could also find themselves awake during surgery. This occurrence is known as anesthesia awareness. The condition of anesthesia awareness (waking up) during surgery, means the patient can recall their surroundings, or an event related to the surgery, while under general anesthesia. In an event where a patient is awake during a surgical procedure, pain is an inconclusive outcome although it has been proven that most patients who have this condition usually don't have any pain or feel a slight, indistinguishable amount of pain. People who have experienced awareness under anesthesia report different levels of awareness. Some people have brief, vague recollections. Others remember a specific moment of surgery or their surroundings. In some cases, people recall a feeling of pressure. (Wilson, 2018) However, the chances of having anesthesia awareness are very rare. In only one or two of every 1,000 medical procedures involving general anesthesia — a patient may become aware or conscious.

Pros/Cons of Anesthetics

While the benefits of anesthesia in surgery continue to become the primary approach to major operations, there is a list of advantages and disadvantages of anesthetics , listed in this chapter. Many would argue that anesthetics is just like any other narcotic drug that numbs the users' mind and pain receptors. Some disadvantages of general anesthesia are that it may cause side effects, such as nausea, vomiting, headache and a delay in the return of normal memory functioning. (Wilson, 2018) In contrast to the advantages of anesthesia, some patients under anesthesia could succumb to lingering effects of sickness, and retention of normal memory. It should be mentioned that these side effects of anesthetics are just a temporary lag from consciousness. These disadvantages of anesthesia are not permanent for patients who feel the lingering effects of post-surgery. Now, the pros of anesthesia explain why it is such an effective approach to surgical procedures. The most obvious advantage is the elimination of the sensory capacity to feel pain during the surgical procedure, which might otherwise be unbearable. This is not only beneficial to the patient, but also to the surgeon, who would otherwise have a hard time dealing with the body's physiological response to stress. This response could cause significant morbidity and mortality if not pre-emptively dealt with by general anesthesia. Amnesia is necessary for reducing and/ or eliminating intra-operative recall, because the average person is not able to withstand the thought of being cut up or cut into, despite not feeling it or seeing it. This experience could subsequently be a source of intensely unpleasant memories, although it is rare for patients to awaken during the surgical procedure. The advantages outweigh the disadvantages of anesthetics in everyday surgeries. The idea of patients sleeping while surgeons operate on them dramatically benefits both parties, which enables the confidence in administering anesthesia for a wide variety of medical procedures. With the advantages of anesthetics, other medical fields such as dental care use anesthetics for surgical procedures like extraction of teeth, implantation of new teeth, and molar crowns. Everyday uses of anesthetics for surgeries benefit many different fields that require the patient to become temporarily immobilized and less receptive to pain to successfully and safely complete the surgical procedure.

The History of Anesthetics

Furthermore, with the advantages and disadvantages of modern Anesthetics, the historical timeline of how anesthesia came to be was a long and treacherous process. Many experiments and observations by several surgeons and dentists contributed to the creation of modern anesthesia. In Scotland, 1847, obstetrician Professor James Y. Simpson started giving women chloroform to ease the pain of childbirth. "Chloroform quickly becomes a popular anesthetic for surgery and dental procedures as well," Chloroform was discovered independently in 1831 by USA's Samuel Guthrie, France's Eugène Soubeiran, and Germany's Justus von Liebig. (Harrah, 2015) The use of chloroform as an anesthetic was the earliest account of a Doctor who wished to operate on unconscious patients. From the late 18th century into the 1840s, physicians and chemists experimented with agents such as nitrous oxide, ether, carbon dioxide, and other chemicals without success. In an era before the adoption of daily dental hygiene and fluoride treatments, excruciating tooth extractions were an all too common part of the human experience.

Consequently, dentists joined physicians and surgeons in the Holy Grail-like search for safe and effective substances to conquer operative pain. (Harrah, 2015) The discovery of modern anesthetics through experimentation inspired Dr. William Morton (mentioned earlier) to continue further experiments with nitrous oxide, including a demonstration at Harvard Medical School in 1845 that failed to completely squelch the pain of a student submitting to a tooth-pulling, thus publicly humiliating the dentist. It was that very moment when Morton grew an obsession to create a substance that would relieve patients from their pain and undergo surgical procedures without the painful experience along with it. During the summer of 1846, Morton purchased bottles of the stuff from his local chemist and began exposing himself and a menagerie of pets to ether fumes. Satisfied with its safety and reliability, he began using ether on his dental patients. Morton used sulfuric ether to anesthetize a man who needed surgery to remove a vascular tumour from his neck, according to "The Painful Story Behind Modern Anesthesia" by Dr. Howard Markel on PBS.org. Surgeon John Warren performed the procedure on patient Glenn Abbott. The success of John Warren's procedure on Glenn Abbott, confirms Dr. Morton's hypothesis surrounding ether fumes. William T.G. Morton called his creation Letheon, named after the Lethe River of Greek mythology, noted for its waters that helped erase "painful memories." (Harrah, 2015) The historical development of modern Anesthesia through Dr. Morton's discoveries has influenced the following years of modern medicine. To this day, the everyday use of anesthesia for surgeries stemmed from the experiments from Dr. Morton and Professor James Y. Simpson, which changed the landscape of medical procedures.

Why Anesthesia is Primarily Used in Surgeries?

Extending ideas mentioned earlier, anesthesia used as a form of medical treatment that prevents patients from feeling pain during and after surgery is one primary reason why it is used frequently in everyday surgeries. Doctors tend to use anesthesia on patients due to its ability to temporarily immobilize patients without lingering effects of pain and discombobulation. The intent of anesthetics for doctors is to work in a less stressful environment without the concern of the patients' health and well-being during the procedure. This means that using anesthetics in everyday surgeries allows doctors to work on unconscious patients without the stress of damage control and possible painful encounters when a patient is conscious when the procedures is being carried out. Everyday surgeries with the use of local, regional, and general anesthetics are the pinnacle of modern medicine. Since its discovery, an estimate of 40 million doses of anesthesia is administered to patients in the United States every year. (Wilson, 2018) If you were to calculate an estimate of how many times anesthesia is used for everyday surgeries in a year, about 110 thousand patients are administered anesthesia before surgery. Looking upon statistics, anesthesia is used daily for medical procedures, and it seems that the administration of anesthetics will continue to increase. The sole reason why anesthesia is widely used by a variety of medical fields is for purposes of numbing and temporarily suppressing pain receptors during the process of surgery. Whether the surgery is major or minor, anesthesia is used to properly execute delicate procedures under the impression that the patient will not feel any kinds of pain while they are under the influence of anesthesia. Although anesthesia is the primary approach for most medical procedures, it is also a proposed option for some patients. Many have argued that the administration of anesthesia is harmful because once administered, the patient will quickly doze off into a deep slumber. However, cases where patients awaken during the procedure experience minor side effects and relatively no pain. According to Family medicine of the Cleveland Health Clinic, "Patients who undergo surgery with the use of anesthesia could, and potentially experience 'Twilight Sedation', which allows the patient to sleep harmlessly without the concern of awakening and experience excruciating pain" (Troianos, 2020) Minor side effects of anesthesia consist nausea, sore throat, and mild pain from the place of incision, which is a rare temporary experience that some patients would come across. Take into consideration that patients should be under the impression that nothing wrong will happen during the procedure. It is entirely up to the doctor to manage the stress and overwhelming emotions that patients are susceptible to before a medical surgery. In everyday surgery, the purpose of anesthesia is to temporarily immobilize the patient, relieving tremendous amounts of pain throughout the procedure. General, regional, and local anesthesia will continue to be the primary approach to most surgical procedures.

Conclusion/Final Thoughts

Anesthesia used in everyday surgeries is a representation of an innovative contribution to modern medicine. Since Dr. Morton's experiments with ether, medical advancements with the development of anesthesia continues to change the landscape of surgical procedures. Many are quick to assume that Anesthesia is an option when approaching surgeries; in retrospect anesthetics is the easiest and most safe approach to any form of surgery. Regardless of it being a major or minor surgery, anesthesia is the main course of action for everyday surgeries. According to Adam C Adler of Medscape Journal explains anesthetics. He states, "An anesthetized patient can be thought of as being in a controlled, reversible state of unconsciousness. Anesthesia enables a patient to tolerate surgical procedures that would otherwise inflict unbearable pain, potentiate extreme physiologic exacerbations, and result in unpleasant memories." (Adler, 2018) Anesthesia at the end of the day is the appropriate course of action for any sort of surgery. From a historical context, the earliest forms of anesthetics were used as a temporary sedative for patients to perform surgery without further complications. Since then, anesthetics is widely used as a temporary sedative and a medicated pain killer for surgery patients. Back when anesthetics had just become part of routine surgery, doctors who administered them knew very little about how they worked, according to the National Institute of General Medical Sciences (NIGMS). Today, it is believed that anesthetics disrupt nerve signals by targeting specific protein molecules inside nerve cell membranes. As scientists continue to learn more about anesthesia, these drugs will only become more effective, says the NIGMS. (Dallas, 2019) Now, every day about 60,000 patients undergo all types of surgery and other medical procedures with the help of these pain-relieving drugs, according to the National Institutes of Health. There's no doubt that anesthesia — whether inhaled as a gas or injected into your bloodstream by a highly trained doctor, dentist, or nurse anesthetist — has enabled millions of people to receive medical treatments that lead to longer and healthier lives. Anesthetics of all forms will always be the medical advancement that changed approaches to surgeries in modern medicine. It is important to understand that anesthetics is the most impactful medical contribution to any medical field.

Local, Regional, and General Anesthesia

By Chitrini Tandon

Anesthesia is given to help provide the patient with comfort and to keep surgeries, medical procedures and tests pain-free (ASA, 2021). As an overview, anesthesia works by temporarily blocking sensory/pain signals the brain centers receive from the nerves (John Hopkins Medicine, 2021). In the human body the peripheral nerves connect the spinal cord to the rest of the body (John Hopkins Medicine, 2021). There are four main categories of anesthesia which are commonly used during surgery and other procedures, these include general anesthesia, local anesthesia, regional anesthesia and sedation or "monitored anesthesia care"(UCLA Health). This chapter focuses on three of these categories: local, regional and general anesthesia. Sometimes, patients may choose which type of anesthesia will be used on them during the procedure (UCLA Health). Before the start of the procedure the physician anesthesiologist will discuss the types of anesthesia that are appropriate and safe to use during the specific procedure and the different options available to the patient (UCLA Health). Side effects vary according to the type of anesthesia that is used but they are usually not detrimental to the patient's health. Also, risks are usually not caused by the anesthesia used but rather by the procedure and/or the patient's previous health history. Anesthesia can be provided by physicians (anesthesiologists), nurse anesthetists, dentists, oral surgeons and anesthesiologist assistants, each of these providers have different levels of training and anesthesiologists receive the most training (Whitlock & Dhingra, 2020).

Before the anesthesiologist can administer any type of anesthetic there must be a plan made. The administrator will gather information on the patient's physical condition, medical history, lifestyle, and medications (John Hopkins Medicine, 2021). Some of the important things they need to know before deciding on the type of anesthetic are if the patient has had any reaction to previous anesthetics, if the patient is taking any current herbal supplements (may cause changes in heart rate and blood pressure), if there are any known allergies (to both food and/or drugs), recent and current prescriptions and use of over-the-counter medication, cigarette smoking and alcohol use (can have strong effects on the body), and lastly, use of other drugs (such as marijuana, cocaine or amphetamines) (John Hopkins Medicine, 2021). Typically before receiving anesthesia patients avoid eating and drinking for eight hours prior to the procedure, quit smoking and taking herbal supplements, do not take Viagra® or other medication for erectile dysfunction for the 24 hours leading to the medical procedure and some forms of blood pressure medications (John Hopkins Medicine, 2021).

Local Anesthesia

Local anesthesia is a term that describes medication such as lidocaine which is injected into the body or applied as a cream and is used to numb a small area (UCLA Health). It is used alone to provide sufficient pain relief for a small amount of procedure such as filling in a dental cavity or stitching a deep cut (UCLA Health). Local anesthesia is typically a one-time use (ASA, 2021). This type of anesthesia is applied to block pain perception which is transmitted to the brain through peripheral nerve fibres (Guilding, 2019). Additionally, local anesthesia is not effective in inflamed tissues (Guilding, 2019). There are two main subfamilies of local anesthesia that are used clinically; ester-linked local anesthesia and amide-linked local anesthesia (Guilding, 2019). It can also be used with sedation during minor outpatient surgery (UCLA Health). Local anesthesia may be used at the end of a procedure to give additional pain relief during the patients' recovery (UCLA Health). Side effects and complications caused by this type of anesthesia are often minor (ASA, 2021). The patient may feel a bit of soreness at the site of injection or in rare instances have an allergic reaction to the anesthesia (ASA, 2021).

There are specifically five administration methods for local anesthesia; topical, infiltration, peripheral nerve block, central nerve block and intravenous regional anaesthesia. With topical administration, a high concentration of the anesthesia is applied and allowed to slowly penetrate through the skin or mucous membrane (Guilding, 2019). Infiltration is when the anesthesia is injected intradermally or subcutaneously, this technique is effective and quicker than topical application (Guilding, 2019). The most common injected local anesthesia is lidocaine (Guilding, 2019). In comparison, in peripheral nerve block, the local anesthesia is injected around the nerve trunk and central nerve block is when it is injected near the spinal cord (Guilding, 2019). Lastly, intravenous regional anaesthesia is when a tourniquet is used to slow down the diffusion of the anesthesia beyond the site of administration, and is often used to manipulate bones in limb fractures or more minor surgeries (Guilding, 2019).

Regional Anesthesia

Regional anesthesia is used to make a specific area of the body numb to prevent the patient from experiencing pain (UCLA Health). This type of anesthesia will stop sensation to the area of the body on which the medical procedure is being performed on. Anesthesiologists inject regional anesthesia near the specific cluster of nerves which are responsible for providing sensation to the area (UCLA Health). Regional anesthesia can also be delivered through a catheter which is a small tube (ASA, 2021). This does not mean that the patient will be completely awake during the procedure, some patients may choose to receive sedation to allow them to relax and doze off during the procedure (UCLA Health). This type of anesthesia can be used in combination with general anesthesia for bigger surgeries such as on the chest or abdomen (UCLA Health). One advantage of using this type of anesthesia is that less opioid pain medication is required after the procedure (UCLA Health).

Two common types of regional anesthesia include spinal and epidural anesthesia and it is common to use either of the two types during childbirth or orthopedic procedures (for example total knee or total hip replacement procedures) (UCLA Health). Epidurals are administered in the back and the medication is sent to the cerebrospinal fluid through the fine needle which is administered to the spinal sac (Whitlock & Dhingra, 2020). Epidurals provide continuous pain relief and there are no side effects to its use (Whitlock & Dhingra, 2020). If the epidural is being used for a chest or abdominal surgery then it is placed higher up the back in order to numb the chest and abdominal areas (John Hopkins Medicine, 2021). Spinal anesthetic is used for the lower abdominal, pelvic, rectal and lower extremity surgery (John Hopkins Medicine, 2021). This type is administered by injecting a single dose in an area surrounding the spinal cord and numbs the lower body (John Hopkins Medicine, 2021). This type is commonly used for lower extremities of orthopedic procedures (John Hopkins Medicine, 2021). Commonly after surgeries on the chest or abdomen or after general anesthesia use, an epidural catheter may be left in the area of the procedure to allow for continued pain relief after a surgery (UCLA Health). Another example of regional anesthesia is a nerve block, this type can provide pain relief to a small area such as an arm or a leg and examples include a femoral nerve block (blocking sensation to the thigh and knee) or brachial plexus block (blocking sensation to the shoulder and arm) (UCLA Health). Regional anesthesia is relatively safe and usually doesn't have complications or side effects (ASA, 2021).

Some side effects of using regional anesthesia include having an allergic reaction, bleeding around the spine, issues with urination, blood pressure dropping, infection in the patient's spine, nerve damage, seizures and severe headaches (Whitlock & Dhingra, 2020). Side effects such as nerve damage and seizures are rare and any concerns should be discussed with the doctor beforehand (Whitlock & Dhingra, 2020).

General Anesthesia

This category of anesthesia is the most common one that most people think of when they hear the word "anesthesia" (UCLA Health). General anesthesia is given for major operations such as heart surgery or cancer treatment procedures (ASA, 2021). These surgeries are often life-saving and life-changing (ASA, 2021). General anesthesia may be used if the procedure takes a long time, results in a large amount of blood loss, the body is exposed to a cold environment or if it affects the patient's breathing (for example chest and upper abdominal surgery)

(Mayo Clinic, 2020). The drugs used as general anesthetics are CNS depressants that can be induced and terminated quickly in comparison to other conventional sedative-hypnotics (Trevor et al., 2015). Modern anesthetics act rapidly and there are four stages of anesthesia: stage 1: analgesia, stage 2: disinhibition, stage 3: surgical anesthesia, and stage 4: medullary depression (Trevor et al., 2015). Under general anesthesia the patient is unconscious and has no awareness or sensation and different medications can be used during general anesthesia (UCLA Health). A breathing tube or mask can be used to provide anesthetic gases or vapors and an IV can be used to provide medication for sleep, relaxing muscles and treating pain (UCLA Health). Some examples of general anesthesia which are inhaled are gas (nitrous oxide) and volatile liquids (halothane) (Trevor et al., 2015). Some examples of intravenous forms of general anesthesia include dissociative (ketamine), opioids (fentanyl), benzodiazepines (midazolam), and miscellaneous (propofol and etomidate) (Trevor et al., 2015). After administration, the patient will be unconscious and body functions will slow down or need help in order to work properly (ASA, 2021). For example, a tube may be placed in the patient's throat to help them breathe (ASA, 2021). Additionally, the patient's heart rate, blood pressure, breathing and other vitals are monitored by the physician anesthesiologist to ensure they are normal and steady while the patient is unconscious (ASA, 2021). After the procedure the physician anesthesiologist then reverses the medication to help the patient regain consciousness and also monitors breathing, circulation and oxygen levels (ASA, 2021).

Overall this type of anesthesia is relatively safe, most complications arise due to the type of procedure or due to the patient's general physical health rather than due to the anesthesia that is used (Mayo Clinic, 2020). Patients who are older in age or have previous medical conditions and those undergoing longer/more difficult procedures are more likely to experience symptoms such as postoperative confusion, pneumonia, stroke, and/or have a heart attack (May Clinic, 2020). Postoperative cognitive dysfunction (confusion) is commonly referred to as "brain-fog" and can lead to learning problems and long-term memory loss (Whitlock & Dhingra, 2020). Some conditions which may increase the patient's risk of complications includes; smoking, seizures, obesity, diabetes, history of heavy alcohol use, and drug allergies among others (Mayo Clinic, 2020).

There are a few side effects that patients might experience from general anesthesia. One of the most frequent side effects is drowsiness after the procedure or surgery. (UCLA Health) The drowsiness typically goes away after the first hour or two after the surgery (UCLA Health). Other side effects include a sore throat from the tube in the patient's throat, chills or nausea (ASA, 2021). It is important to ensure that the physician knows of any history of motion sickness or nausea prior to the procedure so adjustments to medication can be made to prevent nausea afterwards (UCLA Health). Side effects may worsen as the effects of the anesthesia wear off and it might take a day or two for the effects to completely leave the body's system (ASA, 2021). It is rare to experience a serious reaction to general anesthesia but if it does occur there are emergency medications to treat the reaction and vitals are monitored (UCLA Health). Two of the more serious side effects include malignant hyperthermia and breathing problems. Malignant hyperthermia causes a fever, muscle concentrations and can cause death, patients who have previously experienced this or have had a heatstroke are at a higher risk (Whitlock & Dhingra, 2020). Breathing problems can be caused by the patient's throat closing up during surgery and make it more difficult for the patient to regain consciousness and/or breathe normally after the procedure, one risk of this side effect is obstructive sleep apnea (Whitlock & Dhingra, 2020).

Stages

There are four stages of anesthesia; induction, excitement stage, surgical anesthesia and overdose (Weatherspoon, 2018). Stage 1 is induction, this occurs between administration of the anesthetic and the loss of consciousness (Weatherspoon, 2018). The patient will move from analgesia without amnesia to analgesia with amnesia (Weatherspoon, 2018). The second stage is the excitement stage, after losing consciousness this period represents excited and delirious activity (Weatherspoon, 2018). The patient's heart rate and breathing become erratic, there is pupil dilation, nausea, and breath-holding may happen (Weatherspoon, 2018). During this stage there is a risk of choking and vomiting and modern medicine works to minimize the time spent in this stage (Weatherspoon, 2018). Next is stage three, surgical anesthesia where muscles relax, vomiting stops and breathing depresses (Weatherspoon, 2018). Additionally, eye movements will slow and then cease meaning the patient is now ready to operate on (Weatherspoon, 2018). The last stage is stage 4 or overdose, this is when too much medication has been given and leads to brain stem or medullary suppression (Weatherspoon, 2018). This stage might lead to respiratory and/or cardiovascular collapse (Weatherspoon, 2018).

Conclusion

Anesthesia is used to provide a patient with comfort during surgeries and to keep procedures and tests pain free. The four types of anesthesia are general, local, regional and sedation or "monitored anesthesia care". Anesthesia works by temporarily blocking pain signals to the brain. Some examples of those that can give you anesthesia are dentists, anesthesiologists and nurse anesthetists. Before the start of a procedure the administrator will have an interview with a patient to learn more about their history and to develop a plan. The patient may have the option to choose which type of anesthesia they would like to receive. During the procedure the anesthesiologist will monitor the patient's vitals to ensure everything runs smoothly. Local anesthesia typically has no down time while recovery from general and regional anesthesia takes longer. Side effects also vary among the different categories of anesthesia but generally they are temporary and non-life threatening. It is important for a patient to let the health care worker know of any potential risk factors to ensure the correct form of anesthesia is given.

The steps you take after a procedure in relation to anesthesia vary by the type of anesthesia that has been administered. For local anesthesia the patient can return to work and most activities right after the treatment, unless specified by the healthcare worker (Cleveland Clinic, 2020). But, for general and regional anesthesia recovery will take longer (Cleveland Clinic, 2020). Some of the things patients will require is: to have someone to drive them home, rest for the remainder of the day, not drive or operate equipment for 24 hours, no consumption of alcohol for 24 hours, only take medications and supplements approved by the physician and avoid making important or legal decisions for 24 hours (Cleveland Clinic, 2020).

Common Anesthetics Today

Brianna Bedran

There are significant differences in the processes of common anesthetic procedures compared to their first developments. Primitive techniques of anesthesia at the dawn of civilization involved applying pressure on a nerve trunk or artery for temporary loss of sensibility (Leak, 1925, pg. 804). Previous techniques of anesthesia also involved the use of chloroform anesthesia, and even hypnotics, which both proved to be unsuccessful (Leak, 1925, pg. 310-320). Over time and through trial and error, involving unexplainable deaths from certain procedures and frightened doctors and patients, the medical field has made significant developments from these primitive techniques. As a result of these important developments in the medical field since the B.C era, if one saw their surgeon practicing these outdated techniques, this would surely cause worry.

Luckily, common anesthetics and their procedures today involve much more regulation and important safety precautions that must be adhered to. Despite these developments, there are still concerns about anesthetics and their procedures. The development of important safety regulations in anesthetics does not address the additional impact of the chemicals used on our environment. Additionally, infusion rate and the accuracy of monitors of common anesthetics today still require further development. With the help of additional sources, this chapter explores processes and the science behind common anesthetics today and future changes for consideration.

Anesthetic Safety Regulations

Thanks to the World Federation of Societies of Anesthesiologists (WFSA) and World Health Organization (WHO), minimum international safety standards have been implemented for medical practices to ensure these unexplainable deaths and errors in procedures are limited. These specific standards were first introduced in 1992 by the organizations (Kim, et al., 2020, 513). The most common standards mentioned by Yong-Hee Park and Tae-Yop Kim further our understanding of regulations and guidelines in regular anesthesia practice.

Anesthesiologists
As an anesthesia provider, one must be trained to understand the standards recognized and enforced by each country. At any point, anesthesia should ideally be administered and supervised by a specialist in anesthesia and pain medicine when possible. Additionally, consistent communication and cooperation in the operating room and other medical procedures is encouraged, and if not necessary, for a safe procedure with anesthesia.

Facilities and equipment
As doctors performing anesthetics today receive help from monitors, the appropriate facilities and equipment should be

available in the area where anesthesia and recovery are taking place. Just as important is training and safe management of the equipment, which should be conducted on a regular basis.

Drugs, Intravenous infusion and Monitoring
Medications must be labeled. In addition, supplementary oxygen therapy is necessary in all patients undergoing general anesthesia or deep sedation. This is also important for standard monitoring practices which include pulse and respiratory rate, as well as persistent oxygen saturation.

Essential Anesthesia Protocol
It is critical that anesthesia and pain medicine specialists evaluate the patient's condition before the operation. It is the specialist's responsibility for the management during the operation, transfer to the recovery room after the operation, and handing it over to the responsible medical personnel. Patients that have undergone general anesthesia, sedation, or local anesthesia should receive recovery after procedures in a well-maintained and safe recovery space. (Kim, et al., 2020, pg. 514-516).
Our developments in anesthesia safety considerations regulate the internal operations of the procedures. However, Hina Gadani Arun Vyas explains that there are additional impacts that have yet to be seriously considered, such as the effects of commonly used anesthetics on the environment.

Chemical Gasses of Modern Anesthesia

Greenhouse gases include: water vapor, carbon dioxide (CO_2), methane (CH_4), nitrous oxide (N_2O), halogenated fluorocarbons (HCFCs), ozone (O_3), perfluorinated carbons (PFCs), and hydrofluorocarbons (HFCs). The anesthetic agents currently used in the medical field are eruptive halogenated ethers and the common carrier gas nitrous oxide are also known to be dangerous greenhouse gases. As under 5% of delivered halogenated anesthetic are actually being metab-olized by the patient, most of the anesthetics, which are also dangerous greenhouse gases, are emitted to the atmosphere from the source of operation with each procedure.

The halogenated ethers sevoflurane and desflurane are increasingly replacing isoflurane. Sevoflurane (2, 2, 2-trifluoro-1-(trifluoromethyl) ethyl ether), also called fluoro-methyl, is a halogenated ether used for induction and maintenance of general anesthesia. Together with desflurane, it is replacing isoflurane and halothane in modern anesthesiology practice. After desflurane it is the volatile anesthetic with the fastest onset and offset (Gadani, et al., 2011). Nitrous oxide (N_2O) is a colorless, non-flammable gas, more well known as laughing gas due its common and surprisingly gladenning effects, but is used for the purpose of anesthetic and analgesic effects. The gases exhaled by the patient are very similar to those administered by the anesthetist. Often, these anesthetics often are vented out of the building as medical waste gases. These organic anesthetic gases stay dormant in the atmosphere where they can be as harmful as greenhouse gases.

On average, the composition of the waste gases is estimated to be (Gadani, et al., 2011)

> Oxygen 25-30%,
> Nitrogen 60-65%,
> Nitrous oxide 5-10%,
> Volatile halocarbon 0.1-0.5%

Results from The Lund University Hospital demonstrate that the chemical agent N_2O stands for practically 100% of the climate change potential. Although this may have the lowest global warming potential factor out of the four anesthetic gases, the consumed volume of N_2O significantly outweighs the volumes used of the other gases. In the Lund University studies, climate impact from the use of anesthetic gases was compared with the climate impact of energy use. Lund University Hospital used 37 000 MWh of electricity and 50 332 MWh of district heating in 2006. Climate impact of the anesthetic gases corresponds to about one-third of the climate impact emanating from energy use (Gadani, et al., 2011).

Thus, when choosing an anesthetic, it is important to consider the aspects of environmental responsibility. These considerations should not just take global warming into account, but the additional impacts of climate change. Gadani explains that N_2O has a long atmospheric lifetime of about 150 years with a strong warming potential of over 300 times stronger than CO_2, making this a dangerous and effective player in global warming and the destruction of the ozone layer (Gadani, et al., 2011).

Common practices of anesthetics today should consider these environmental impacts. Gadani and other contributors explain that further safety procedures to cover these external impacts should involve the use of scavenging systems and waste reduction techniques of employing capture technology that uses canisters to collect wasted anesthetics. Common anesthetics face a new challenge that invokes them to introduce new ideas. These new ideas should change ingrained behavior and create the desire among staff, patients, suppliers and volunteers to attempt something different. Additionally, any new ideas that address environmental concerns should involve advice from environmental teams, as well as medical gas and equipment suppliers (Gadani, et al., 2011).

Induction Process of Common Anesthetics

The process of induction can be performed intravenously with a constant rate or intermittent infusion, with the use of a target-controlled infusion system, commonly known as a TCI system. TCI systems administer drugs dependent on a variety of medical factors of the patient. The system takes into account age, weight, height, and gender and continuously simulates the drug concentration in the body, and controls drug administration either by effect-site or plasma concentration targeting (Ferreira, et al., 2019). In simpler terms, an anesthesiologists should decide on the drug target concentration for a patient based on their specific simulated expected response, and with that information administer the necessary dose. TCI systems are a product of the importance of con-trolling the level of anesthesia during routine administration. Despite any basic administration standards we previously mentioned, every patient's need is subjective and the TCI system takes these differences into account by administering the proper dose-dependent on the factors of age, weight, etc. However, the depths of anaesthesia have yet to be clearly defined, thus adequate anesthetic control remains rather ambiguous (Ferreira, et al., 2019).As a result, a variety of methods for the assessment of the hypnotic compartment of anaesthesia has been developed.

Loss of consciousness as a goal of certain procedures occurs during the induction process of general anesthesia practices. It is important to detect and be sure of the moment the patient loses consciousness, as identifying the exact moment will determine the individual response of each patient to the hypnotic. Determining this exact moment also provides relative information to guide the proper infusion rate necessary to maintain a sufficient level of anesthesia, delivering effective care (Ferreira, et al., 2019).

The rate of infusion is crucial because it prevents intraoperative awareness and overdose, two dangerous and certainly preventable problems that catch the attention of clinicians, and these associated risks can often alarm patients. Intraoperative awareness occurs if a patient under general anaesthesia regains consciousness (Ferreira, et al., 2019). Typically, this is a result of insufficient hypnotics, and is a frightening experience that causes long term morbidity in some patients. However, it should be noted that the chances of experiencing intraoperative awareness is relatively low. Cases of intraoperative awareness as concluded by large multicentre studies, were approximately 1–2 per 1000 cases (Ferreira, et al., 2019). Another alarming impact of improper rate of infusion is overdose. Overdose of anesthesia occurs if a patient receives an overly necessary amount of a hypnotic drug, which is why we use TCI systems. This can lead to severe brain stem or medullary depression, which can further result in respiratory and cardiovascular collapse (Ferreira, et al., 2019). These impacts can be fatal.

The importance of administering hypnotics slowly to prevent anesthetic overdose is widely accepted, encouraged, and a common anesthetic practice nowadays to prevent these fatal impacts. Studies have demonstrated that the required doses for a patient undergoing anaesthesia are affected by variation in the rate of injection. Conducting a slow infusion rate results in longer induction time, but requires a lower total dose, and reduces the chances of experiencing apnoea and loss of blood pressure (Ferreira, et al., 2019).

Considering the current risks of improper induction explained above, A.L Ferreira suggests that anaesthesia monitoring should include both subjective and objective methods. The subjective methods in this context are based on movement and autonomic response to stimuli, as well as relying on the advice and experience of the anaesthesiologist. Objective methods rely on the accuracy of a monitor (Ferreira, et al., 2019). Commercial depth-of-anaesthesia monitors often use a dimensionless monotonic index as a measure of the depth of anaesthesia. The dimensionless monotonic index typically ranges from 100, which indicates an awake state, to 0, which indicates a deep coma. (Ferreria, et al., 2019). There is a large variety of monitors to assess the differences in patients and anaesthesia indexes, such as "System Monitor (BIS Monitor; Covidien, USA), Entropy Module (GE Healthcare, USA), Narcotrend (MonitorTechnik, Germany), Patient State Index Monitor, SEDLine (Masimo, USA), Cerebral State Monitor (Danmeter, Denmark), loC-View Monitor (Aircraft Medical, Barcelona, Spain), qCon (Quantium Medical, Spain) and lastly AEP Monitor (Danmeter, Denmark)" (Ferreira, et al., 2019).

However, despite their useful information and assistance, these monitors may fail in identifying the exact moment consciousness is lost, which we have described is a crucial moment of procedures. Monitors face computation delays, difficulties in separating the different electrical signals produced by the body, and the large interindividual variability of the monitor indices suggest monitors are beneficial when it comes to indicating the evolution of the patient during the procedure, but fail to identify the moment of loss of consciousness. Studies show that combining depth-of-anaesthesia monitors with the information provided by the clinical signs reduced the incidence of intraoperative awakening and over-dosing (Ferreira, et al., 2019). There is still need for a system that detects the exact moment in which the patient loses consciousness, however. By identifying this moment during the induction phase of general anesthesia, this will determine the dose of hypnotics required by each patient, and will provide significant information to guide the necessary infusion rate to maintain an appropriate and adequate level of anaesthesia. Ferreira and other contributors suggest this can open the door to automated systems based solely on the patient's state of consciousness, making important advances in the field of anaesthesia (Ferreira, et al., 2019).

Conclusion

The significant developments in anesthetics compared to its first operations demonstrate the importance of regulation and safety standards in common anesthetics. Anesthetic practice today involves enforced policies and advanced technology to help with procedures, when its first developments were more of trial and error with a variation of results. Patients are also more aware of the associated risks with anesthesia thanks to any google search, applying more pressure on the medical field for near perfection. However, perfection will always be difficult, if not impossible to achieve, and this chapter by no means scrutinizes the inaccuracies and negative impacts of anesthetic practice. It is worth noting, however, that development is needed in the induction process of common anesthesia and the use of the associated chemical agents. Researchers suggest an accurate induction process indicating the exact moment of loss of consciousness and a proper induction rate is a huge step for the medical field towards further reducing the risks of intraoperative awareness and overdose. Additionally, reassessing the chemicals used and how to properly dispose of their waste from procedures rather than it be vented in the air is highly recommended. Common anesthetic practices today have made a long journey from first operations and will continue to be reassessed and require development.

Interactions with the Nervous System

By Camryn Kabir-Bahk

The interactions which occur between anesthetics and the nervous system are essential to ensuring the functionality of anesthesiology. This chapter discusses how anesthetics work with the nervous system. The nervous system has the daunting task of regulating, controlling and communicating all of the activities that occur in the body. For example, it regulates and controls breathing, movement, metabolism, and much more. The nervous system does this by using two primary components: the central nervous system and the peripheral nervous system.

Components of the Nervous System:

The Central Nervous System (CNS) is critical in coordinating activities in the body based on the sensory information that it receives (Cherry, 2020). The CNS is composed of the spinal cord and brain (Skaggs, 2013). The brain controls both mental (memory) and physical (movement, awareness, sensory) functions. The brain has a left and right hemisphere divided into four different lobes, which are interconnected: frontal, occipital, parietal and temporal lobes (Cherry, 2020). Each of these lobes has a distinct function but works with each other to coordinate necessary activity. The frontal lobes are related to higher-level thinking, cognition, language and voluntary movements (Cherry, 2020). The occipital lobes are related to controlling visual processes, and the parietal lobes are tasked with processing sensory information (Cherry, 2020). Lastly, the temporal lobes are vital in coordinating hearing, sound and the formation of new memories (Cherry, 2020). The brain stem connects to the brain by the base of the temporal lobes. The bottom of the brain stem then connects to the spinal cord. The spinal cord can be thought of as a midpoint between the brain and the nerves located throughout the rest of the body. The spinal cord transmits messages brought to it from the nerves located throughout the body and directs it to the brain for the activity to be carried out. The interaction between the spinal cord and nerves is essential in integrating the peripheral and central nervous systems.

The Peripheral Nervous System

Small nerves are attached to the spinal cord extend to many regions of the body and make up the peripheral nervous system (PNS) (Skaggs, 2013). The PNS connects the CNS to the rest of the body. The brain and spinal cord communicate with other regions of the body via the PNS. The messages which get transmitted back and forth allow the body to carry out functions or react to stimuli in the environment (Cherry, 2020). The PNS is composed of two components; the autonomic nervous system and the somatic nervous system. The autonomic nervous system controls involuntary functions, such as breathing, heartbeat, or digestion (Cherry, 2020). These are vital functions that are maintained under the influence of anesthetics. The somatic nervous system communicates sensory and motor information to and from the CNS using two types of neurons; motor and sensory neurons. Motor neurons, also known as efferent neurons, convey signals from the CNS to muscle fibres located within the body (Cherry, 2020). Sensory neurons or afferent neurons carry signals from nerves located outside of the CNS and transmit them to the brain and spinal cord (Cherry, 2020). The integration of these two neurons keeps activity in the body under regulation.

Neurons

There are multiple ways to send and receive information throughout the nervous system (Skaggs, 2013). Certain chemicals known as hormones are released into the body, typically through the bloodstream. Hormones travelling around the body will look for their target. Once the target is found, the hormone will bind to receptor proteins on the cell's surface and carry out the function the hormone was sent to do. The diffusion of hormones into the body is advantageous since it can cover a wide range of areas in the body (Skaggs, 2013). However, this process is lacking specificity (Skaggs, 2013). Instead, neural signalling is much more specific, precise and faster than the release of hormones (Skaggs, 2013).

Neural signalling makes use of neurons and neurotransmitters to communicate a signal. A neuron is a specialized cell that can communicate with other cells by synapses (Skaggs, 2013). Neurons are the primary cell used in cell and neural signalling when communicating messages across the nervous system. A neuron or nerve cell comprises three major parts; the cell body, axon and dendrites. Each component of a neuron is critical to carrying out a signal. Neurons can be described as long cells. The dendrites and axons are on either side of the cell body (Lodish, 1970). Dendrites resemble branch-like structures and are essential in receiving signals at their synapses, which is the specific location for signal receiving (Lodish, 1970). Neural signals are then shot down the cell body towards the other end of the neuron, where the axons are located. These signals are electrochemical waves known as an action potential (Skaggs, 2013). Action potentials are sent from an axon terminal to the next synapses located on the dendrite of a different neuron (Skaggs, 2013). Synapses are vital in enabling neural signals to be sent throughout the body. In fact, there are hundreds of different synapses within the body. Typically, synapses are divided into two categories; chemical or electrical (Skaggs, 2013). Electrical synapses use the passage of ions between neurons to communicate signals (Skaggs, 2013). While electrical synapses can be useful, chemical synapses have a wide range of functions and are frequently used (Skaggs, 2013). When a signal is released from a cell, that cell is called presynaptic. The cell which receives the signal is called postsynaptic (Skaggs, 2013).

The area around where a synapse is located has an abundance of synaptic vesicles. These vesicles are filled with neurotransmitters (Lodish, 1970). Neurotransmitters are diverse and each type of neurotransmitter has a different function (Lodish, 1970). A rise in the level of $Ca2+$ occurs when an action potential has reached the axon terminal and is ready to be sent to the next cell (Lodish, 1970). A higher level of $Ca2+$ causes the vesicles to bind to the plasma membrane of the presynaptic cell and release the neurotransmitter (Lodish 1970). The neurotransmitters diffuse across the synaptic cleft to the postsynaptic cell (Lodish, 1970). Once the neurotransmitters have reached the postsynaptic cell, they bind to receptors located on the surface of the cell. The ion permeability of the postsynaptic cell's plasma membrane changes in response to the binding of the neurotransmitters. The change in ion permeability affects the plasma membrane's electrical potential. This, coupled with the binding of a neurotransmitter to its paired receptor, carries out the neural signal (Lodish, 1970). Signals can be inhibitory or excitatory. Inhibitory neurotransmission suppresses an action potential from firing and excitatory neurotransmission increases the chance of an action potential firing (Skaggs, 2013). Without this process, cell signals, whether inhibitory or excitatory would not occur.

How anesthetics interact with CNS

General anesthesia is one of the most common types of anesthesia used today. It is used typically before extensive medical procedures. However, despite the use of general anesthesia for hundreds of years, the mechanism it uses is not fully understood (Son, 2010). The state in which general anesthesia inflicts upon a patient differs based on the concentration of anesthetic used.

General anesthesia has been found to have significant effects on the central nervous system. It functions by promoting inhibitory neurotransmission and minimizing excitatory neurotransmission across the CNS (Son, 2010). The interaction between a neurotransmitter and its receptor is likely the target that anesthetics attempt to reach. Changing this interaction will change the function of the signal that was supposed to be carried out and regulate an anesthetic state. When a patient is put under general anesthesia, they can undergo various stages of being in an anesthetic state (Son, 2010). However, the neural pathways and receptors that regulate unconsciousness under anesthesia will differ from those regulating immobility under anesthesia.

Therefore, anesthetics will function on specific molecular targets and work in the areas of the brain that are responsible for certain behavioural responses under anesthesia (Son, 2010). Although there is not enough evidence to prove the association between all regions of the brain and a behaviour associated with general anesthesia, some relationships have been found (Son, 2010). The effect of amnesia under general anesthesia has been found to be associated with the hippocampus (Son, 2010). Sedation and unconsciousness under general anesthesia are closely related to the neocortex and thalamus (Son, 2010). After basic neuroimaging of the brain under anesthetics, many images displayed that the thalamus was a key region anesthetics targeted to influence unconsciousness (Alkire & Miller, 2005). A possible reason for this is that anesthetics work to induce a neuronal hyperpolarization block in regions of the thalamus, prompting unconsciousness (Alkire & Miller, 2005).

Ion channels are an interesting protein to look at in order to understand some of the interactions that general anesthetics have with the nervous system. Ion channel receptors are located on the plasma membrane of some cells (Alberts, 1970). Ion channels are transmembrane proteins that mediate the passage of certain types of ions. They are located near synapses play a large role in interacting with neurotransmitters and permitting a signal (Alberts, 1970). There is a great deal of interest in ion channels and the possibility that they are one of the functional sites for general anesthesia (Son, 2010).

Although, there are hundreds of different types of ion channels found in the body, the γ-aminobutyric acid type A (GABAA) subunit receptor has been found to have a vital role in the functional sites of general anesthetics (Son, 2010). GABA is the most abundant inhibitory neurotransmitter found in the brain and about a third of all synapses are related to the GABA neurotransmitter (Son, 2010). GABAA receptors are chloride-permeable ligand-gated ion channels (Son, 2010). The activation of these receptors is followed by a rise in the level of chloride found in the cell membrane and the hyper-polarization of the cell membrane (Son, 2010). This will cause an inhibitory post-synaptic potential (de Leon & Tadi, 2020). GABA will transfer information to GABAA receptors by creating inhibitory postsynaptic currents (Son, 2010). General anesthetics act on GABAA receptors by enhancing the inhibitory function of GABA neurotransmitters (Son, 2010). Some general anesthetics have even been able to activate GABAA receptors without GABA being present (Son, 2010). In the past few years, there has been more evidence that has revealed a lasting type of tonic (slow) inhibition in many areas of the brain. Tonic inhibition is caused by tonic currents produced when low amounts of GABA act on high affinity extrasynaptic GABAA receptors (Son, 2010). The excitability of neurons and its ability to process information has been shown to be controlled by tonic conductance. General anesthetics have been found to promote the effect that tonic currents (Son, 2010). This discovery indicates that a major functional site of general anesthetics are extrasynaptic GABAA receptors. Many different subunits for GABA receptors exist. However in the case of the functional sites of volatile anesthetics, it has been found that the α1, β1 and β3 subunits of GABAA receptors are closely associated with these sites (Mihic et al., 1997). Inhibiting aspects of the nervous system are closely linked with various subunits of the GABAA receptor (Son, 2010). For instance, the tonic currents that are produced in the hippocampus are associated with the function of memory and cognition under general anesthesia (Son, 2010). Isoflurane is volatile general anesthetic which can enhance the tonic currents in the hippocampus (Son, 2010). These currents act on the subunit α5 GABAA receptor at a higher capacity due to the effects of isoflurane. This interaction is considered one of the mechanisms that general anesthetics use to prompt amnesia while a patient is under anesthesia (Son, 2010). Other anesthetics such as propofol and etomidate can prompt the same results.

Many ion channels other than GABAA receptors exist and can be affected by anesthetics. Glycine receptors have become a candidate for another functional site of anesthesia. Glycine receptors are found mostly along the spinal cord and the brain stem (Avila et al., 2013). They enhance the same inhibitory functions as GABAA receptors (Son, 2010). Therefore, they interact with general anesthesia using a mechanism similar to that of GABAA receptors. However, instead of affecting amnesia, glycine receptors have been found to have a strong effect on the lack of response the body will have to a painful stimulus (Son, 2010).

Local anesthetics

More is known about how local anesthetics work with the nervous system. Local anesthetics are drugs that numb a specific region of the body. Local anesthetics are typically used in medical or dental procedures (Becker & Reed, 2012). They work by blocking neural connections which will stop the patient from feeling a painful sensation. This is done by blocking the movement of large amounts of sodium ions through ion channels in the plasma membrane (Becker & Reed, 2012). Without the presence of anesthetics, sodium ion channels in their resting state will deny the entry of sodium ions until the stimulation of a neuron (Becker & Reed, 2012). Once a neuron is stimulated, the channel activates and opens to allow sodium ions to pass and initiate the depolarization across the membrane (Becker & Reed, 2012). After the movement of sodium ions, the channel will deactivate and quickly close, stopping ions from moving (Becker & Reed, 2012). The neuron will then carry on the signal to the next cell. The ion channels attached to the neuron which sent the signal will then go back to its resting state. Local anesthetics work to block this process from occurring and stop the patient from feeling pain. Local anesthetics have a high affinity for receptors on sodium ion channels that are activated instead of when they are in the resting state (Becker & Reed, 2012). So, neurons that are quickly firing off signals are very vulnerable to a local anesthetic. Lidocaine is a widely used local anesthetic that uses this mechanism to inhibit pain response.

A very common type of local anesthetic is epidural. Epidural is used to help people during labour manage the pain that comes with childbirth (Institute for Quality and Efficiency in Health-care, 2018). A small amount of epidural is injected into the epidural space of the spine (Institute for Quality and Efficiency in Healthcare, 2018). The epidural space is filled with fluid and surrounds the lower area of the spine. Epidural works to block certain nerves on the spinal cord from sending pain signals from the spinal cord to the brain (Institute for Quality and Efficiency in Healthcare, 2018). This is a very effective method of relieving pain sensation in the lower half of the body for patients in labour.

A lot is still unknown about the nature of general anesthetics. The assumption that anesthetics do not cause long-term negative effects because they are reversible has been taken for granted. In the last few years, it has become increasingly evident that anesthetics can affect cellular processes, protein synthesis, and gene expression (Perouansky et al., 2009). Evidence generated from research on anesthesia-induced neurotoxicity on rats suggests that exposure to general anesthesia at a young age can prompt neural communication damage (Wu et al., 2019). This is likely caused by widespread neuroapoptosis (programmed death of brain cells) (Wu et al., 2019).

One of the major pathological indications of Alzheimer's disease is the hyperphosphorylation of the tau protein (Wu et al., 2019). Tau is a protein used to stimulate the assembly of microtubules in brain cells (Gong & Iqbal, 2008). Tau is a phosphoprotein and when it becomes hyperphosphorylated, tau is unable to regulate the assembly of microtubules (Gong & Iqbal, 2008). This leads to tangling and tau buildup in a neuron, which inhibits the ability of a neuron to send a signal. In an experiment done with mice that did not have any cognitive defects, it was found that repeated exposure to anesthetics such as sevoflurane and propofol leads to tau hyperphosphorylation in the hippocampus (Wu et al., 2019). In addition, the mice then participated in the Morris Water Maze test. The results indicated that the mice experienced significant damage to their spatial memory (Wu et al., 2019). These are the results of only one experiment. However, there are strong indications that ageing brains exposed to anesthesia can have lasting negative effects on cognitive abilities (Wu et al., 2019).

Although the effects of anesthesia wear off for many patients after a few hours, there is still a strong possibility that anesthetics can have detrimental effects on the brain and nervous system. Neurotoxicity, neuroapoptosis and Alzheimer's disease or only a few of the researched issues that may arise with the use of anesthetics. Although this may be concerning, changing the use of anesthetics for clinical practice is not necessary yet (Perouansky et al., 2009). More research needs to be done to have a better understanding of the effects that anesthetics can have on the nervous system.

Anesthesia Awareness

By Yi Yang Fei

In February 2020, a video clip of a violinist's performance gained attention in the news industry (Reuters, 2020). It was not an average performance one would expect. Distinct from her regular roles in orchestra and choral societies, the musician expressed her musicality as a patient during a brain tumour removal surgery (Reuters, 2020). The procedure was deliberately selected to preserve the patient's ability to play violin, as the affected region in the right frontal lobe controls fine movement on the left hand (Reuters, 2020). Through brain mapping, the surgical team carefully avoided damaging the brain regions activated during performance and ultimately removed more than 90% of the tumour (Reuters, 2020). The distinct contrast between the instrument's soothing tune and the precise operations behind the surgical drape undoubtedly creates a unique sight (Reuters, 2020).

Nevertheless, this is not a new technique for the field of brain surgery. Two years prior, Piai et al. (2018) published a detailed case report describing a similar approach for their patient. In their case, the tumour infiltrated the left supplementary motor area, which enables sequencing of movements and is thus involved in motor skills required for performing (Piai et al., 2018). They noted only one musical mistake intraoperatively and were able to remove 95% of the tumour (Piai et al., 2018). The authors further reported that the patient resumed activity two weeks after the surgery and even returned to playing in the orchestra as soon as six weeks into recovery, thereby success-fully preserving abilities for music performance (Piai et al., 2018). The procedure is scientifically known as awake cran-iotomy (Piai et al., 2018). It was introduced first as a surgical intervention for epilepsy, but it has been subsequently adapted for managing certain tumors, aneurysms, and disease-specific needs such as deep brain stimulation (Piccioni & Fanzio, 2008). In particular, awake craniotomy has often been used for lesions in eloquent brain structures that support crucial cognitive functions such as motor, speech, or senses (Eseonu et al., 2017; Martino et al., 2011). By pairing electrocorticography with the patient's active response to elec-trical stimulation, the procedure is able to guide the surgeon in making critical intraoperative decisions that are advanta-geous for patient outcome (Piccioni & Fanzio, 2008).

However, unsurprisingly, anesthetic management remains a challenging aspect of such surgical procedures (Garavaglia et al., 2014). The anesthesiologist must induce adequate sedation and analgesia while maintaining stable conditions for both respiratory control and awake mapping (Eseonu et al., 2017; Garavaglia et al., 2014). As such, to prioritize patient safety, awake craniotomy is not recommended for patients with comorbidities such as pulmonary or psychiatric disorders due to concern for airway obstruction or other detrimental effects in the event of oversedation (Garavaglia et al., 2014). However, the potentially beneficial patient outcome from undergoing awake craniotomy is still an incentive to explore this choice (Garavaglia et al., 2014). Garavaglia et al.'s (2014) study reported successful operations on 10 patients who would traditionally be considered high-risk and thus be recommended against awake craniotomy. The procedure involved the use of bupivacaine-based scalp nerve block and dexmedetomidine while avoiding airway manipulation (Garavaglia et al., 2014). This can be considered as a form of monitored anesthesia care (MAC), where sedation manages pain and agitation without affecting conscious response to commands or invasive instruments in the airway (Eseonu et al., 2017). In contrast, the asleep-awake-asleep (AAA) technique requires the use of instruments such as endotracheal tubes to secure the airway before and after conscious cortical mapping of the patient (Eseonu et al., 2017). Therefore, either MAC or AAA, along with the option to recommend against awake craniotomy, may be considered in the surgical team's preoperative evaluation to ultimately reduce psychophysical stress of the patient (Eseonu et al., 2017; Piccioni & Fanzio, 2008).

Anesthetic procedures in awake craniotomy aim to preserve consciousness for cortical mapping intraoperatively. However, how would awareness affect patients in the case that they were unintended to be awake in the first place? Directed by Joby Harold (2007), the film Awake describes a patient who remains alert yet paralyzed during a heart transplant, thereby unable to express his pain to pause the procedure (Galley & Hall, 2008). Contrary to the awe brought by the video of the musician undergoing awake craniotomy, this film raised fear and concern for patient safety from both organizations and individuals seeking medical advice (Galley & Hall, 2008; Orser et al., 2007). Broadcasting and news organizations also interviewed survivors of anesthesia awareness who experienced long-term psychological complications, which further induces fear for audiences who have an upcoming surgery planned (Galley & Hall, 2008). This fear is not a new phenomenon. Long before the film's release, intraoperative awareness and postoperative pain were found to be the two most common sources of anxiety in a cohort of 247 patients receiving general anesthesia for dental procedures (McCleane & Cooper, 1990). In addition, Samuelsson et al. 's (2007) study found that the presence of acute emotions such as fear, panic, and helplessness during awareness episodes was statistically correlated with development of postoperative psychological symptoms such as anxiety, nightmares, and flashbacks. In their study, 33% or 15 out of 46 patients reported having psychological symptoms after the awareness episode (Samuelsson et al., 2007). Duration of such postoperative symptoms can range from three weeks to several years, and additional psychiatric care would likely be needed for severe cases such as those who develop post-traumatic stress disorder (PTSD) (Bruchas et al., 2011; Sandin et al., 2000; Samuelsson et al., 2007).

In literature, the phenomenon of anesthesia awareness is named as accidental awareness during general anaesthesia (AAGA) (Pandit et al., 2014). It describes the unintended ability of patients to explicitly recall intraoperative experiences during general anesthesia through either spontaneous reporting or direct questioning (Tasbihgou et al., 2018). On a wider scope, however, accidental awareness during anesthesia (AAGA) is a rare occurrence with an incidence between 1 or 2 cases per 1000 patients under general anesthesia (Orser et al., 2007; Pandit et al., 2014; Sebel et al., 2004). For cases of awareness, not all experience pain. Other sensations include sounds, somatic sensations, or emotions (Leslie & Davidson, 2010). Among a cohort with 46 cases of awareness during general anesthesia, Samuelsson et al. (2007) found 43% or 20 patients who experienced pain and 65% or 30 patients who described acute emotions in their aware states. However, these estimates may vary between studies and subpopulations. For instance, Sebel et al. (2004) suggests that the incidence of awareness with recall after general anesthesia may increase to 0.36% from 0.13% if cases of possible awareness are considered along with confirmed awareness cases. Certain risk factors are also associated with higher incidences of the event due to variations in patient characteristics, surgical procedures, and anesthetic techniques (Chung, 2014). Specific risk factors will be elaborated on later in this chapter.

Nevertheless, the associated psychological sequelae are not restricted to awareness during general anesthesia alone (Kent et al., 2013). Recall from a previous chapter that anesthesia can be local, regional, or general. Scalp block, which was described previously as a component of anesthetic care in awake craniotomy surgeries, is an example of local anesthesia which often involves the use of bupivacaine (Piccioni & Fanzio, 2008). Although complete amnesia may occur during sedation and regional anesthesia, it is expected that regional anesthesia leaves the patient arousable with possible painless auditory recall of intraoperative events (Kent et al., 2013; Orser et al., 2008). In comparison, awareness is not intended when the patient is under general anesthesia, which can be inferred from the term "accidental" (Kent et al., 2013; Pandit et al., 2014). However, such expectations originate from the provider's perspective (Kent et al., 2013). For patients receiving anesthesia, the boundary between the different types of anesthetics is less clear, possibly due to failure of informed preoperative consent or miscommunication between provider and patient (Kent et al., 2013). Rather than pain or awareness events themselves, such differences in expectations from either the provider's or the patient's perspective may be a source of distress (Mashour et al., 2009). Kent et al.'s (2013) study also found comparable persistence and presence of psychological sequelae between those who received regional anesthetics and those who received general anesthesia. This phenomenon demonstrates the importance of communication between physician and patient in regards to expectations from anesthesia in order to mitigate psychological distress (Kent et al., 2013).

Cause and Consequences of Anesthesia Awareness

In essence, AAGA is a consequence of an imbalance between the administered dosage of anesthetic and the required amount of anesthetic for the patient under general anesthesia (Leslie & Davidson, 2010). There are four broad categories that can result in insufficient anesthetic effects (Orser et al., 2007). First, there may be unexpected variations in dose requirements between patients (Orser et al., 2007). It has been suggested that genetic differences may contribute to heterogeneity in the effect of anesthetic drugs on protein channels, which may make certain patients more susceptible to AAGA (Pandit et al., 2014). Indeed, a previous awareness episode is a risk factor for AAGA, and a case with family history of AAGA has been noted (Pandit et al., 2014). Second, the patient may have a known complication that makes them physiologically intolerant to a sufficient dosage, such as cases with poor cardiac functions or hypovolemia (Orser et al., 2007). Patients may also have concurrent interventions that mask an increased dose requirement (Orser et al., 2007). Lastly, equipment malfunction or misjudgement from the anesthesiologist will result in insufficient dosage of anesthetics as well (Leslie & Davidson, 2010).

There are three main goals of general anesthesia: hypnosis, where the patient is expected to be unconscious; analgesia, which mitigates or avoids physiological response to pain; and amnesia, where intraoperative events are not remembered postoperatively (Tasbihgou et al., 2018; Wang et al., 2012). Amnesia can further be divided into anterograde, when an amnestic drug is administered prior to amnesia, and retrograde, when a drug is administered after an event to suppress memory formation and thus rescue the patient from recall of the event (American Society of Anesthesiologists, 2006). The expression of recall can also differ between explicit memory, when the patient is able to recall specific events during the awareness episode, and implicit memory, when behavioural change is observed in the patient without recall of events that influenced the change (American Society of Anesthesiologists, 2006). As such, AAGA can be confirmed through both direct questioning and spontaneous reporting, and it represents an incidence of inadequate anesthesia administration (Sury, 2016). The Modified Brice questionnaire, for instance, asks the patient a series of six questions about their experience, such as if they recall events before or after the surgery, if they dreamed of anything, or if anything was unpleasant (Tasbihgou et al., 2018). Nevertheless, the possibility of false memories may be induced by certain interview protocols, especially when leading prompts were used that could convince the patient of something that did not actually occur (Cook et al., 2014). Historically, postoperative interview was considered as the gold standard to assess adequacy of anesthetics on its own (Wang et al., 2012). This was based on the incorrect assumption that consciousness must correlate with postoperative recall of events (Wang et al., 2012). Currently, it is agreed that intraoperative states exist on a spectrum, including binary conditions such as conscious or unconscious, as well as presence or absence of response to command (Wang et al., 2012). In addition, postoperative states also present a spectrum of conditions (Wang et al., 2012). The patient may have explicit or implicit recall, and the memories may or may not include pain or distress (Wang et al., 2012). As well, psychological sequelae may be present or absent, such as PTSD or nightmares (Wang et al., 2012). Notably, memories of AAGA may not emerge immediately after surgery (Cook et al., 2014).

The ability of anesthetic or narcotic drugs to induce amnesic effects, however, creates an ethical concern. Specifically, regardless of the ability to induce amnesia or prevent recall of events, it would be unethical to allow the patient to experience pain or emotional distress during the surgical procedure (Wang et al., 2012). Additional challenges are posed when drugs with neuromuscular blockade effects are induced to limit mobility of the patient or induce paralysis (Cook et al., 2014; Tasbihgou et al., 2018). When the patient is paralyzed due to administration of neuromuscular blocking drugs, it may not be possible to assess consciousness due to the patient's inability to initiate purposeful movements to stimuli (American Society of Anesthesiologists, 2006). Furthermore, the incidence of awareness is found to be higher when neuro-muscular blocking drugs were used than when they are not used (Pandit et al., 2014; Sandin et al., 2000). As distress and longer-term harm are also more likely when the patient experiences paralysis during AAGA regardless of pain perception, use of neuromuscular blocking drugs should be either minimized or accompanied with intraoperative monitoring (Cook et al., 2014; Tasbihgou et al., 2018). The Isolated Forearm Technique (IFT) uses such an approach, where one arm is isolated from the effect of neuromuscular blocking drug in circulation using an inflated cuff (Pandit et al., 2015). As such, the patient's consciousness can be assessed upon command to move the un-paralysed hand or arm, and dosage of anesthetics can be increased if necessary (Pandit et al., 2015).

Patient Care and Management of AAGA

Considering the consequences of AAGA on patient outcomes, the American Society of Anesthesiologists (2006) prepared a practice advisory report for providers to assist in decision making during patient care. In particular, there are several possible time points for interventions. Prior to the operation, the provider must evaluate medical history or exams to determine whether the patients are at risk of AAGA due to risk factors proposed in literature (American Society of Anesthesiologists, 2006). The patients should be informed of the possibility of intraoperative awareness and other expectations or perception during the surgery (American Society of Anesthesiologists, 2006). During the pre-induction phase of anesthesia, functionality of drug delivery systems should be checked to prevent AAGA due to equipment malfunction (American Society of Anesthesiologists, 2006). During the operation, intraoperative monitoring may occur either through clinical techniques, such as assessing movements or commands, or through brain electrical activity monitors (American Society of Anesthesiologists, 2006). These may include electroencephalograms (EEGs) which provide an index, such as the Bispectral Index, that is scaled between zero to 100 depending on the state of consciousness (American Society of Anesthesiologists, 2006; Myles et al., 2004). Intraoperative monitoring should, however, rely on more than one modalities to ensure minimization of the possibility of AAGA (American Society of Anesthesiologists, 2006). Lastly, if consciousness is determined, the provider may inject benzodiazepine intraoperatively and assess AAGA postoperatively (American Society of Anesthesiologists, 2006). If an AAGA case is detected, the provider must communicate with the patient to find potential reasons for such awareness and offer postoperative counseling or support (American Society of Anesthesiologists, 2006).

Can Hypnosis Replace Anesthesia?

By Cassandra Van Drunen-LaChanse

While hypnosis has garnered a bad reputation due to its past association with stage performance and charlatanism, it is making a comeback in the medical field (Holden, 2012). Hypnosis is a unique concept that has been heavily researched as a tool for pain relief. This technique can be used to create a day-dreaming like effect on a patient (Ketterhagen et al., 2002). More specifically, hypnosis can be defined as the creation of a subjective state within a patient under which changes in terms of memory and perception can occur through suggestion (Wobst, 2007). However, an imperative stipulation of hypnosis is willing participation (Ketterhagen et al., 2002). Hypnosis is composed of three parts: absorption, dissociation, and susceptibility (Vanhaudenhuyse et al., 2013). Absorption refers to the inclination to be "fully involved in a perceptual, imaginative, or ideational experience" (Vanhaudenhuyse et al., 2013). Conversely, dissociation is indicative of becoming mentally separate from one or more components of an experience that under normal circumstances would be processed together (Vanhaudenhuyse et al., 2013). Finally, susceptibility involves one's ability to respond to social cues, which can cause an individual or patient to have an increased predisposition to agree with hypnotic instructions or suggestions (Vanhaudenhuyse et al., 2013). In the past, hypnosis has been frequently used in many medical and psychiatric settings, including pain management, depression, and post-traumatic stress disorder (PTSD) (Cozzolino et al., 2020). While as early as the 19th century hypnosis was the only form of anesthesia used, the discovery and implementation of general anesthetic drugs such as diethyl ether caused the use of hypnosis to become restricted in the field of surgery (Cozzolino et al., 2020). However, the use of hypnosis in surgical settings made a temporary resurgence during World War II due to drug shortages (Cozzolino et al., 2020). Now, in the twenty-first century, the use of hypnosis to replace or work adjunctly with classical anesthetics is continuing to be explored and implemented.

The Impact of Hypnosis on the Body

While the concept of hypnosis has been explained, the question still remains: How does hypnosis work? The neuro-physiology of hypnosis on a patient has been studied to attempt to explain this phenomenon. As far back as 1969, it was found that while under hypnosis, metabolic activation occurred within specific cortical regions of the brain (Maquet et al., 1999). These regions included the occipital, parietal, precentral, premotor, and ventrolateral prefrontal cortices on the left hemisphere of the brain as well as the occipital and anterior cingulate cortices on the right hemisphere (Maquet et al., 1999). Additionally, a decreased activation was observed in the precuneus, bilateral temporal, medial prefrontal and right premotor cortices (Maquet et al., 1999). These results were understandable when compared to a previous study that regional cerebral blood flow was increased by 16% in individuals who had undergone hypnosis, specifically in the occipital and right temporal regions (Vanhaudenhuyse et al., 2013). Additionally, a later function magnetic resonance imaging (MRI) study discovered that there was a difference in brain structure size between individuals who were low and highly hypnotizable (Vanhaudenhuyse et al., 2013). The highly hypnotizable subjects were found to have a 32% larger rostrum of the corpus callosum than those with low hypnotizability (Vanhaudenhuyse et al., 2013). This region of the brain is associated with allocation of attention as well as movement of information within the prefrontal cortices (Vanhaudenhuyse et al., 2013). The impact of hypnosis on the human body continues to be studied and understood.

The Different Hypnosis Techniques

Various specialists use different techniques to induce hypnosis. The quintessential technique used to produce hypnosis involves direct suggestions of relaxation, imagining a "special or safe space", or suggestions of pain relief and reductions in anxiety (Drouet & Chedeau, 2016). An additional technique is known as Ericksonian Hypnosis, which was created by psychiatrist Milton H. Erickson (Lankton, 2016). As opposed to the previously mentioned traditional form of hypnosis, Ericksonian Hypnosis relies on indirect suggestion (Lankton 2016). This method of hypnosis often involved a form of storytelling (sometimes referred to as a therapeutic metaphor) instead of directly suggesting specific behaviors to minimize conscious resistance to hypnosis (Lankton, 2016). Another hypnotic technique known as hypnopraxia was first introduced and published in 2005 (Drouet & Chedeau, 2016). Originating from Eriksonian hypnosis, the act of hypnopraxia relies on a specialist withdrawing all judgement and knowledge they believe to have on the patient (Drouet &

Chedeau, 2016). This allows the specialist to be able to "accept the patient's experience of himself, as well as that of the outside world" (Drouet & Chedeau, 2016). In simpler terms, hynopraxia is the act working with the patient's action "in the moment" by taking note of the patient's verbal structure, body movements and their own current experience of reality (Drouet & Chedeau, 2016). Hypnopraxia is often not referred to as a technique but rather as accompanying a patient that is conducted by the patient themselves through a specialist (Drouet & Chedeau, 2016). This subset of hypnosis was found to be successful in a small study of five patients undergoing surgical procedures who all stated that they were satisfied with the results after the procedure (Drouet & Chedeau, 2016). It is important to note that two of these patients received sufentanil (a pain relief drug) and local anesthetic alongside the use of hypnopraxia (Drouet & Chedeau, 2016). While many forms of hypnosis exist, the form that is most effective is dependent on the patient being treated. It is made most apparent by Erickson that "[a] variety of individual approaches may be employed ... To this end, some subjects need to feel themselves dominated by the hypnotist, others want to be coaxed of persuaded, some wish to go into the trance as a result of joint cooperative endeavor, and there are those who wish, or more properly need, to be overwhelmed by a wealth of repetitious suggestions, guiding every response they make" (Lankton, 2020).

Hypnosis in Pediatrics

In modern society, many medical fields have studied the potential use of hypnosis as either a replacement to anesthesia or in addition to anesthesia. One of these fields is pediatrics. Back in 2009, a case study was performed on a thirteen year old boy with severe pulmonary arterial hypertension (Von Ungern-Sternberg & Habre, 2009). This patient, who was described as "severely anxious", needed surgery to implant a Broviac® central line so he could receive a constant infusion of prostacyclin intravenously (Von Ungern-Sternberg & Habre, 2009). Since this patient was at high risk for general anesthesia, his surgical team suggested the use of Erikson-style hypnosis based on positive suggestions (Von Ungern-Sternberg & Habre, 2009). The team performed a hypnosis trial before his surgery date to ensure the patient was accustomed to the process (Von Ungern-Sternberg & Habre, 2009). On the day of the surgery, hypnosis was induced approximately 15 minutes prior to the procedure (Von Ungern-Sternberg & Habre, 2009). Aside from some nausea at the start of the procedure (for which 2.5 mg of ondansetron was administered), all of the potential stimulating or painful events that could have occurred (including the feeling of cold during disinfection, stinging during infiltration of local anesthetic, subcutaneous tunneling of the Broviac® catheter, etc.) were included in the hypnosis in various forms, leading the 2.5 hour surgery to be described as "uneventful" (Von Ungern-Sternberg & Habre, 2009). The patient said they had no memory of what happened in the surgery after his hypnosis was induced and complained of only slight pain 6 hours after his surgery at his incision sites, for which paracetamol was administered (Von Ungern-Sternberg & Habre, 2009). Overall, this study hypnosis could be a "good alternative to general anesthesia", if general anesthesia could not be used (Von Ungern-Sternberg & Habre, 2009). However, as this is only discussing one patient, more research would be required to strengthen these claims.

Since this case study, other extensive studies have been conducted to determine the validity of hypnosis being used as an anesthetic. A later Canadian report investigated the use of hypnosis as a pre-, peri-, and post-anesthesia (Kuttner, 2012). It has previously been determined that 60% of children and

80% of adolescents experience anxiety before surgery (Kuttner, 2012). Therefore, it is important to find ways to battle this common anxiety as these pre-anesthetic fears may cause repercussions on a patient's recovery (Kuttner, 2012). The article discusses a randomized study of 50 children (aged 2-11 years old) that were separated into a midazolam or hypnosis group (Kuttner, 2012). Using a modified Yale Preoperative Anxiety Scale, specialists found that there were less children in the hypnosis group that were anxious than in the midazolam group (39% v.s. 68%) (Kuttner, 2012). When entering post-operative care, the hypnosis group was found to have displayed less behavioural distress then the midazolam group on the first day (30% v.s. 62%) and continued onto the seventh day (26% v.s. 59%) (Kuttner, 2012). Additionally, after performing a research analysis, it was found that the use of pediatric periop-erative hypnosis for invasive medical procedures (eg. bone marrow aspirations) was more effective at eliminating discom-fort across all the studies when compared to the control group (Kuttner, 2012). While these results are promising, not all researchers agree with the validity of these claims. A report by Manyande et al. describes the aforementioned hypnosis v.s. midazolam study as having a "very low grade" quality of evidence (Manyande et al., 2015). However, the report claims that hypnosis as well as other non-pharmacological interven-tions to assist with the induction of anesthesia, such as the use of clown doctors or playing video games of the child's choice, could be promising areas of research in the future (Manyande et al., 2015).

Hypnosis in Dentistry

Dentistry is another field of medicine where hypnosis has been tested. However, the rates of success vary across different studies and use. A study conducted at the Johannes Gutenberg

University in Mainz and of University Medicine Mainz involving 34 participants ranging in age from 21-54 years worked to compare the use of hypnosis and local anesthesia to enact dental pain relief (Wolf et al., 2016). This study revealed that the pain threshold when using hypnosis had a mean value of 58.3, whereas the mean pain threshold when using local anesthesia was found to be 79.4 (Wolf et al., 2016). It is interesting, however that while local anesthesia was found to be more effective in dental pain relief, approximately one-quarter of patients stated that hypnosis was their method of choice for pain management while at the dentist (Wolf et al., 2016). The paper concludes that while local anesthesia remains the gold standard treatment option, adjutant use of hypnosis for minor procedures is recommended (Wolf et al., 2016).

Despite the lack of promise for the use of hypnosis in this study, a more recent case study shows a potential important application in the field of dentistry. The case study discusses a female patient who was unable to use local anesthesia for her dental procedure due to a multisystem disorder known as multiple chemical sensitivity (MCS) (Cozzolino et al., 2020). This MCS, otherwise known as environmental illness, sick building syndrome, or idiopathic environmental intolerance, is a medical condition that is still relatively unknown in modern society (Cozzolino et al., 2020). While much about this condition is unknown, after exposure to specific compounds individuals can experience a wide range of symptoms (Cozzolino et al., 2020). Some of these symptoms are as mild as headache, fatigue, itching, and muscular weakness or as severe as respiratory difficulties, auto-immune conditions, anxiety or depression (Cozzolino et al., 2020). A 32-year-old female patient diagnosed with MCS and had a known intolerance to local anesthetics was required to undergo a procedure to remove left inferior third molar in dysodontiasis (Cozzolino et al., 2020). The patient underwent hypnosis anesthesia for 40 minutes to complete the surgery and stated after the fact that she experienced no pain, was satisfied with the procedure, and had vivid memories of each surgical stage (Cozzolino et al., 2020). This study poses a potential research avenue for hypnosis in the medical field. If further patients with MCS were studied, in both dentistry and other medical fields and procedures, hypnosis could potentially be used more extensively for this sub-group of individuals (Cozzolino et al., 2020).

Hypnosis in Cancer Surgery

A final intriguing field in which hypnosis has been studied is in breast cancer care. In a 2019 study, a group of researchers studied the impact of perioperative hypnosedation on post mastectomy care (Lacroix et al., 2019). Forty-two breast cancer patients, ranging in age from 39-75 years old), who underwent a mastectomy surgery were split into two groups: those who received general anesthesia and those who received hypnosedation (Lacroix et al., 2019). The study aimed to determine the incidence of postmastectomy pain syndrome (PMPS) (Lacroix et al., 2019). PMPS is estimated to occur in 20-60% of post-mastectomy patients (Lacroix et al., 2019). While there is no standard definition of PMPS in the medical field, it remains a substantial health care problem for women (Lacroix et al., 2019). The study concluded that there was a significantly lower incidence of PMPS in the hypnosis than in the general anesthesia group (Lacroix et al., 2019). Additionally, there were decreased incidences of decreased shoulder range of motion post-surgery and anxiety (Lacroix et al., 2019). Overall, the study demonstrated the potential benefits of using hypnosis as anesthesia (Lacroix et al., 2019). However, as seen in many other current studies regarding hynosedation, the small sample size causes limitations in generalizability and validity (Lacroix et al., 2019).

General Knowledge of Hypnosis and Cost

While the many positive results that have been reported that using hypnosis as anesthesia sound great, are anesthesia providers ready for hypnosis? A study surveyed various anesthesiologists, nurse anesthetists, as well as interns, residents and fellows with the field of anesthesia to answer this exact question (Stone et al., 2016). Of the 126 individuals surveyed, over 70% rated that their knowledge of hypnosis was either below average or that they had no knowledge (Stone et al., 2016). Additionally, while only 42% of providers agreed or strongly agreed that hypnotherapy had a place in the clinical setting of anesthesia, 83% agreed that positive suggestions should be involved in anesthesia (Stone et al., 2016). Therefore, if and when hypnosis is found to be a beneficial practice in the medical field, knowledge and acceptance of the practice will need to be spread.

In the same report, Stone et al. discussed an interesting positive reason to use hypnosis as anesthesia in health care. The use of hypnosis can lower the cost of various procedures (Stone et al., 2016). For example, it was found that using hypnosis for interventional radiology procedures reduces the cost by $338 per case (Stone et al., 2016). Additionally, in breast cancer surgical patients, it was found that using hypnosis reduced the cost by about $773 per patient, as well as reducing the time in the operating room by nearly 11 minutes (Stone et al., 2016). This intriguing analysis may also have a more significant impact on the healthcare system if hypnosis becomes a more readily used method of anesthesia use.

Conclusion

In conclusion, the concept of using hypnosis is a rich area of modern research. While there have been few strong claims due to small sample sizes or other limitations, many articles believe that, with more research, hypnosis could have a potential place either as a sole anesthesia or adjutant with other local or general anesthesias in certain medical settings. It has been demonstrated that many fields, ranging from pediatrics to dentistry, could benefit from further research and use of this non-pharmacological anesthesia method. As anesthesiologist Elizabeth Rebello stated, if hypersedation may be a better plan in certain settings, "we owe it to our patients to explore this option [hypnotherapy]" (Bruno, 2019).

Narcotics as Anesthetics

Noah Varghese

The topic of anesthesia often goes hand in hand with another group of medications and drugs, narcotics. Narcotics and anesthetics are both used for similar purposes and share a history but are different in other regards such as the mechanism of action and availability. Ultimately, the differences of both types of drugs stem from their similar but differing definitions concerning pain relief. As a reminder, anesthetics are drugs that induce a loss of sensation, although the operational definition of the drug varies within the literature (Nambiar, 2020). Conversely, narcotics are classified as analgesics, which are drugs solely responsible for the loss of pain (Nambiar, 2020). Therefore, anesthetics encompass all the properties of analgesics, but the opposite cannot be said. Furthermore, narcotics are defined as psychoactive analgesics that are derived from or based on opium, which is itself an extract from the juice of the poppy plant (Rosenblum et al., 2008). To better understand why the discussion of narcotics is important concerning the topic of anesthesia, let's explore more about the biochemical properties of opium and its derivatives.

Opium refers to the dried latex found within the seed capsules of the poppy plants ("Opium: Uses, Addiction Treatment & Side Effects", n.d.). It has a rich history and is one of the earliest plants that were cultivated for medicinal value. The drug can be administered in several ways, and each route of administration can induce different effects on the user (Rosenblum et al., 2008). For example, it can be inhaled, which can induce quick but short-lasting effects, or it can be absorbed intravenously, which will instead induce delayed longer-lasting symptoms (Nakhaee et al., 2020). Narcotics primarily work by binding to opioid receptors, which is a general term of receptors found within most organisms, including other vertebrates and even some invertebrates (Rosenblum et al., 2008) (Brownstein, 1993). Some of these opioid receptors are associated with inducing pain relief, which when bound to opium is responsible for the feelings of euphoria (Forget, 2019) (Brownstein, 1993). However, since opium binds to a multitude of other receptors in the body, it is also responsible for a list of other side effects such as nausea, vomiting, respiratory depression, and the most well-known effect: physical dependence (Forget, 2019) (Vella-Brincat & MacLeod, 2007). Not all anesthetics target opioid receptors, but they do target receptors that are often found within the same cell type: cells in the central and peripheral nervous system (Russell et al., 1987) (Brohan & Goudra, 2017). For example, a receptor for propofol, a common general anesthetic, is GABA subunit A, which is an ion channel found within the brain and is responsible for dulling all sensations (Brohan & Goudra, 2017).

Although there are other types of analgesics, narcotics are the predominant type of analgesic that is used in the field of medicine, solely for its effectiveness. Specifically, many other non-narcotic analgesics to achieve the three clinical outcomes of anesthesia: the patient must be unconscious, immobile, and have no control over the autonomic nervous system (Egan, 2019). Opioids can achieve all these outcomes of anesthesia with ease, but the main reason it is used in current anesthesia operations is its remarkable ability to induce the loss of control of the autonomic nervous system (Egan, 2019). Additionally, the rich history of opioids also merits a strong foundation of research behind the formation of its derivatives as well as the already implemented infrastructure to grow said drug. The infrastructure that is being referred to is the large-scale opium farms found in Asia and the large international trade relations that make opium somewhat far more available than most other analgesics. Furthermore, narcotics are a wide class of drugs, and there are many variants, either synthetic or natural, that have different properties (Rosenblum et al., 2008). That being said, opioids are infamously known for their toxic and addictive properties hence why history is riddled with multiple occurrences of the "opium epidemics," a time where a large percentage of deaths can be attributed to opioid overdose (Netherland & Hansen, 2016). These epidemics also fueled or at least related to lots of other political issues, that involved race or poverty, which helped push the agenda that all forms of opiates should be banned (Netherland & Hansen, 2016). Narcotics are therefore controversial since it is debatable if we should use something this toxic and addictive to treat patients. That is why for some time the field of medicine tried to shift away from the use of narcotics as anesthetics for opioid-free anesthesia (Rosenblum et al., 2008). In this chapter, we will explore the relationship between narcotics and anesthetics, determine whether it is appropriate if these drugs can be used interchangeably under certain circumstances. When talking about opium and its place in medicine, it would be ignorant to not consider the history of opium in ancient and modern history, since it explains not only its medicinal roots but also its ties to economy and culture, which is something to consider if are to use narcotics as anesthetics.

Opioid use is not something novel and has been intertwined with medicine and politics for centuries. To better understand whether opioids can be used as a substitute for regular anesthetics, the long history of opioids should be explored further. The first recorded instance of cultivating opioids was in 3400 BC by the Sumerians in Mesopotamia from poppy plants (Rosenblum et al., 2008). Early on in history, there was already a well-established index of the different variety of opioids based on what type of poppy plant it was extracted from (Schiff, 2001). These different juices had slightly different effects such as some inducing more drowsiness or having other euphoric effects. Opium was viewed as a symbol of joy and the knowledge of its cultivation and its effects were passed on to Assyrians, Babylonians, and Egyptians (Brownstein, 1993). This when the spread of opium and its importance in the world started to grow.

What happened in Egypt is one of the first instances in history where opium became part of iconography and was part of the culture and religion (Schiff, 2001). This became noteworthy since, during the 1300s, opium in Egypt was no longer something associated with commoners but instead with people of privilege and power (Schiff, 2001). The only people that could handle opium were those of nobility or those who were linked to their deities and religion. It was incorporated into mythology such as when deities would use opium to treat other ailments such as headaches. Additionally, not only was opium used for medicinal purposes but it was also used for other facets of their daily routine, such as putting infants to sleep and for recreation (even though it was mainly used for religious rituals) (Schiff, 2001). Around this time, opium was also used in surgery to relieve any pain, indicating early on how narcotics fulfilled some of the functions of modern-day anesthetic procedures (History.com Editors, 2017). Opium evolved to be something no longer restricted to simple recreation but also has extended to something more of a symbol.

While Egypt was exploring the use of opium, they were also responsible for spreading the use of opium to other ancient civilizations before 500 AD, including that of Ancient Greece (History.com Editors, 2017). Like Egypt, Greece quickly integrated the use of opium into the rest of its culture, such as with mythology, philosophy, and even in law. For mythology, Homer, who is a well-known author responsible for writing the Iliad and Odyssey, references opium in his works when writing about the Greek deities (Bandyopadhyay, 2019). To further emphasize the symbol opium had in ancient Greece, deities such as Hypnos and Thanatos, who are the gods of sleep and death respectively, were usually surrounded by poppy flowers (Kritikos & Papadaki, 1967). Additionally, Hippocrates, who is considered the father of medicine, praised opium for its healing properties and its ability to induce drowsiness (Schiff, 2001). This ties in with the already existing belief in Greece of how sleep was considered as the best treatment for all ailments, which works well with opioids as a sleep-inducing drug (Schiff, 2001). Although Hippocrates advocated for the drug, there was still debate as to how frequently people should use it given the harmful effects narcotics have (Kritikos & Papadaki, 1967). For example, Diagoras, who was a founder of the Alexandrian Schools, disapproved of Hippocrates' suggestions of using opium for mild ailments (Kritikos & Papadaki, 1967). Therefore, opium epidemics existed even during the times of ancient civilization and were becoming so much of a problem that its regular use had to be questioned and be a source of controversy. But even amongst the controversy, opium served an important role not only in medicine but also in the justice system (Schiff, 2001).

Specifically, Ancient Greece and even Ancient Rome used opium as a means for executing enemies and criminals through an overdose, since it was painless. With this belief, many citizens of Ancient Rome also used opium overdose as a means of suicide given that euthanasia was accepted (Schiff, 2001). By this point, many civilizations took a similar stance to that of Ancient Greece and started to use opium commonly especially in the field of medicine (Schiff, 2001).

Other Ancient civilizations involved with opium distribution include China and India, both of whom are heavily involved with opium production and distribution in the current economy. In both nations, there were recorded instances of where opium was used in surgical procedures just like in the other previously discussed nations as anesthesia. Ancient China and India also integrated opium into their mythology, but it also slowly became a topic of politics and economy. For example, jump forward to 1839, when international relationships were forming and there was the establishment of opium trade routes throughout the world (Schiff, 2001). During this point of time, the Opium Wars took place because of the British empire "weaponizing" opium (Lu et al., 2007). Specifically, opium was heavily restricted in China, and the British capitalized on that opium's addictive nature to push trade between both nations to fuel the British's rapid industrialization (Lu et al., 2007). The reason this was mentioned is to emphasize the power of opium politically but also how many nations, specifically the Chinese government, recognized the harmful health effects of opium to general productivity even though it was recognized as an important drug in the medical field. Around this time, opium use and death have skyrocketed where one-third of deaths were associated with opium overdose in the 1830s (Bandyopadhyay, 2019).

Around the 1800s, the properties of opium started to be investigated to exploit and enhance the properties of the drugs (Eddy, 1957). For example, crude opium from the poppy plant juice was used to create derivatives like that of morphine in 1803, although natural crude opium was still preferred over all the other alternatives (Eddy, 1957). Additionally, as new opioid derivatives were being discovered, two new classes of opioids were formed: synthetic, like fentanyl, and semi-synthetic derivatives, like heroin. Regardless of where it was derived, these narcotic alternatives were always marketed as having less or no addictive properties, which was untrue. As a consequence of this lie, these alternatives would be mistakenly sought out by the public out of the belief that they would induce the same euphoria as conventional opium but with none of the harmful side effects (Eddy, 1957). Eventually, the distribution of opium and the growing physical dependence not only was a problem just found in China but in many other nations, hence why in 1909 the International Opium Commission was founded to decrease the production and importation of opium (Schiff, 2001). This commission would later grow until eventually it was undertaken by the League of Nations and then the United Nations (Schiff, 2001). The public opinion towards opium is strongly negative, even within the medical community, although this will shift as the field of anesthesia changes.

The general opinion of narcotics among the scientific community started to shift as soon as new less harmful narcotics were started to be created. An example of one significant change was the discovery of nalorphine, which serves as an antagonist to the activity of opium (Brownstein, 1993). Nalorphine was discovered in 1942 and it was discovered to reverse opioid overdose, even though it is an opiate derivative. Only a short time later, was another derivative, methadone discovered to induce the same effects of morphine but have fewer addictive properties (Rosenblum et al., 2008). Consequently, it has been used in replacement therapy where addiction to narcotics can be lessened by switching from the original opioid to that of methadone. This eventually led to a shift in perception of narcotics in the science community in the 1990s where opioids were used predominantly to treat chronic pain, which was a condition that was becoming increasingly more frequent (Rosenblum et al., 2008). Chronic pain can emerge from a multitude of illnesses, including that of cancer, hence why narcotics medicinal use has lost some of its stigmas, at least in medicinal practice (Rosenblum et al., 2008).

Opioid use in modern medicine is used solely as an anesthetic or at least as an adjuvant in anesthetic procedures. Although the US Food and Drug Administration has approved the use of narcotics in every phase of surgery, many physicians and surgeons actively avoid narcotics due to potential complications in favour of non-narcotic alternatives (Ferry & Dhanjal, 2021). For example, a common problem with using narcotics even in a controlled medical setting is that it has been associated with increased physical dependence on opium among patients. This is still up for debate since multiple studies like a study in Sweden, have shown that after making methadone more readily available to cancer patients, there was no increase in illicit drug use (Agenas et al., 1982). Therefore, this highlights how the association of addiction with narcotics use is still not well understood and must be investigated further. Another potential consequence of using opioids is the fear that it is responsible for the proliferation of cancer cell lines. This is quite ironic given that opioids are often given to cancer patients given how they often suffer chronic pain (Rosenblum et al., 2008). It is believed that narcotics increase cancer incidence rates since it is found to suppress the immune system (Afsharimani et al., 2011).

Specifically, it was found in one study to be responsible for suppressing innate immune cells from recognizing and stopping the growth of tumour cells, but it also halts the adaptive immune response to produce antibodies that target metastasizing malignancies (Sacerdote et al., 2000). Additionally, many opioid receptors are involved with angiogenesis and cell adhesion, both of which are important for metastasis (Afsharimani et al., 2011). However, it should be mentioned that the idea of opioids being responsible for initiating or proliferating tumours is also up for debate given that nanomolar concentrations of morphine were observed to be pro-apoptotic towards some cancer cells based on cell type. What is clear however is that opioids were shown to be responsible for decreasing the motility of the immune cells, thereby delaying the immune response (Roy et al., 2006). Therefore, many heroin users tend to be susceptible to a list of other illnesses because of a compromised immune system (Roy et al., 2006). Finally, another concern is that some individuals demonstrated anaphylaxis and other allergic reactions to some narcotics like fentanyl (Rojas-Pérez-Ezquerra et al., 2019). With all these concerns regarding narcotic use as anesthesia, its effectiveness as an analgesic for anesthesia is not something to be ignored, hence why there is active research to mitigate these negative consequences.

To overcome the dangers of narcotics many physicians have devised strategies to overcome the difficulties of using the drugs at least in a clinical setting. One strategy that is growing in popularity is the use of a multimodal anesthesia technique, where multiple anesthetics are used simultaneously (Ferry & Dhanjal, 2021). Specifically, this technique involves the use of other anesthetic agents, with each agent only focusing on one of the three clinical outcomes of anesthesia. Opioids in this case are primarily used to induce a loss of control over the autonomic nervous system, while other anesthetics, such as propofol will be used in conjunction. The multimodal anesthesia technique is growing popular given that it requires a smaller dose of all anesthetics in general and thus lowers the chances of any harmful side effects from any of the drugs (Egan & Svensen, 2018). Additionally, most other anesthetics are not as effective as opioids in reducing post-operative pain (Egan & Svensen, 2018). There are drugs such as esmolol and adenosine that achieve a similar function to that of conventional narcotics, however, it is less effective since it requires a larger dose and more expensive equipment (Egan, 2019). Furthermore, there are synergies between different anesthetics, which can accelerate recovery time (Egan & Svensen, 2018). Note this efficacy doesn't apply to all narcotics since morphine is relatively useful in reducing pain but fentanyl is not. There has also been a shift in outlook as to how to handle patient care, in which each patient case would be classified under different pain subtypes (Schwenk & Mariano, 2018). Some pain subtypes include neuropathic, psychogenic, or idiopathic, and all these classifications are assigned based on the type of surgery as well as other factors specific to that of the patient. Different mixtures of anesthetics will be applied based on the subtype, which emphasizes the careful application of narcotics and other medication to minimize side effects (Schwenk & Mariano, 2018).

Regardless of the current opinions, narcotics have shaped the field of medicine and anesthesia and even now are currently being investigated in further detail to minimize the side effects. As mentioned prior the most popular technique for administering narcotics is in conjunction with other anesthetics since opioids are still proven to be one of the best drugs for achieving the 3 clinical outcomes of anesthesia. There is still much to learn about the drug, its interactions with other anesthetics, as well as the existence of better alternatives but what can be said now is narcotics do play an important role in the field of medicine today and probably will continue to be important in the future.

References

Chapter 1: Origins from Natural Sources

A Jewish Virtual Library. (2008, January 12). Abu Bakr Muhammad ibn Zakariya al-Razi (841–926). https:// www.jewishvirtuallibrary.org/abu-bakr-muhammad-ibn-zakariya-al-razi. Ägyptisches Museum und Papyrussammlung. Princess Meritaten offering a mandrake plant to her husband, King Smenkhkare.

Baraka, A., (1982). Historical Aspects of Opium. Middle East J Anaesthesiol, 6, 289-302.

Bates, D., Robinson, W., Jeffery, Charles. (1990). Biology and Utilization of the Cucurbitaceae. Cornell University Press.

Belayneh, A., & Bussa, N. (2014). Ethnomedicinal plants used to treat human ailments in the prehistoric place of Harla and Dengego valleys, Eastern Ethiopia. J Ethnobiology Ethnomedicine, 10(18). https://doi.org/10.1186/1746-4269-10-18

Booth, M. (1996) The discovery of dreams. Opium: A History. London: Simon & Schuster.

Brownstein, M (1993). A brief history of opiates, opioid peptides and opioid receptors. Proceedings of the National

Academy of Sciences of the United States of America. 90(12), 5391–5393.

Burstein, H.J., Gelber, S., Guadagnoli, E., & Weeks, J.C. (1999). Use of Alternative Medicine by Women with Early-Stage Breast Cancer. New England Journal of Medicine, 340(22), 1733-1739. 10.1056/NEJM199906033402206

Carter, A., (1996). Narcosis and nightshade. Br Med J, 313, 1630-1632.

Dams, I., Martin, B., (1996). Cannabis: Pharmacology and Toxicology in animals and humans. Addiction, 91, 1585-1614.

Fritz, K. (2021). The Importance of Rights to the Argument for the Decriminalization of Drugs. The American Journal of Bioethics, 21(4), 46-48. https://doi.org/10.1080/15265161.2021.1891337

Government Central Printing Office. (1894). Indian Hemp Drugs Commission. (1893-1894) Report on Indian Hemp.

Green K. (1998). Marijuana smoking vs cannabinoids for glaucoma therapy. Archives of Ophthalmology, 116(11), 1433–1437. https://doi.org/10.1001/archopht.116.11.1433

Haddad, F., (2003). The Spongia Somnifera. Middle East J Anesthesiol, 17, 321-327.

Health Canada. (2016). A Framework for the Legalization and Regulation of Cannabis in Canada: The Final Report of the Task Force on Cannabis Legalization and Regulation. https://www.canada.ca/en/health-canada/services/drugs-medication/cannabis/laws-regulations/task-force-cannabis-legalization-regulation/framework-legalization-regulation-cannabis-in-canada.html

Heydari, M., Hashempur, M., Zargaran, A. (2013). Medicinal aspects of opium as described in Avicenna's Canon of Medicine. Acta Medico-historica Adriatica, 11(1), 101-112. Information Canada. (1972). Commission of Inquiry into the Non-Medical Use of Drugs (Le Dain Commission). http://publications.gc.ca/collections/collection_2014/sc-hc/H21-5370-2-1-eng.pdf

Juvin, P., Desmonts, J., (2000). The Ancestors of Inhalational anesthesia: The soporific sponges (Xlth-XVIIth centuries), Anesthesiology, 93, 265-269.

Kalant, H. (2001). Medicinal use of cannabis: History and current status. Pain Res Manage, 6(2), 80-91. https://downloads.hindawi.com/journals/prm/2001/469629.pdf

Kalant, OJ. (1972). Report of the Indian Hemp Drugs Commission, 1893-94: A Critical Review. International Journal of Addiction, 7, 77-96.

Kritikos, P., & Papadaki, S. (1967). The early history of the poppy and opium. Journal of the Archaeological Society of Athens.

Lee, M. (2006). The Solanaceae: foods and poisons. J R Coll Physicians Edinb, 36, 162-169.

Lee, M. (2006). The Solanaceae II: The Mandrake (Mandragora offcinarum): In League with the

Devil. J R Coll Physicians Edinb, 36, 278-285.

Magner, L. (1992). A History of Medicine. New York: Marcel Dekker.

Morimoto, S., Kazunari, S., Jun, M., Futoshi, T., Hiroyuki, T., Mariko, A., Masakazu, T.,

Hiroshi, S., Yasuyuki, S., Yukihiro, S., (2001). Morphine Metabolism in the Opium Poppy and Its Possible Physiological Function. Journal of Biological Chemistry. 276(41), 38179–38184. doi:10.1074/jbc.M107105200

Mussema, Y. (2006). A historical overview of traditional medicine practices & policy in Ethiopia. J Ethnobiology Ethnomedicine, 20 (2), 127-134.

Needham, J. (1974). Science and Civilisation in China: Spagyrical discovery and invention: magisteries of gold and immortality. Cambridge University Press.

Needham, J., Ping-Yu, H., & Gwei-djen, L. (1980). Science and Civilization in China: Volume 5, Chemistry and Chemical Technology. Cambridge University Press.

Newmaster, SG; Grguric, M; Shanmughanandhan, D; Ramalingam, S; Ragupathy, S (2013). DNA barcoding detects contamination and substitution in North American herbal products. BMC Medicine, 11(222), doi:10.1186/1741-7015-11-222

Okunade, A. (2002). Ageratum conyzoides L. (Asteraceae). Fitoterapia, 73(1), 1-16. https://doi.org/10.1016/S0367-326X(01)00364-1.

Operational Medicine 2001 Field Medical Service School Student Handbook: Molle medical bag/surgical instrument set. (1999, December 7). https://brooksidepress.org/Products/OperationalMedicine/DATA/operationalmed/Manuals/FMSS/MOLLEMEDICALBAG.htm.

Pennacchio, M., (2010). Uses & Abuses of Plant-Derived Smoke: Its Ethnobotany as Hallucinogen, Perfume, Incense & Medicine. Oxford University Press.

Salguero, C (2009). The Buddhist medicine King in literary context: reconsidering an early medieval example of Indian influence on Chinese medicine and surgery. History of Religions, 48 (3), 183-210. doi:10.1086/598230

Schultes, R., (1970). Random Thoughts and Queries on the Botany of Cannabis. In C. Joyce & S. Curry (Eds.), The Botany and Chemistry of Cannabis (pp. 11-38). London: J & A Churchill.

Small, M. (1962) Oliver Wendell Holmes. New York: Twayne Publishers.

Stewart, A., (2009). A Wicked Plants: The Weed that Killed Lincoln's Mother and Other Botanical Atrocities. Algonquin Books.

Suppan, L., (1918). Mandrake and Mandrake Mannikins, The National Druggist. St. Louis: Henry R. Strong Publishers, 48, 99-102.

Vishal, S., Nutan, S., Prasad, P., (2013). Medicinal Plants from Solanaceae Family. Research J. Pharm. and Tech, 6(2), 143-151.

Webster, G. (1994). Synopsis of the Genera and Suprageneric Taxa of Euphorbiaceae. Annals of the Missouri Botanical Garden, 81, 33-144. doi:10.2307/2399909

World Health Organization. (2011). Quality Control Methods for Herbal Materials. file:///C:/Users/Admin/Downloads/9789241500739_eng.pdf

World Health Organization. (2013). WHO Traditional Medicine Strategy 2014-2023. http://apps.who.int/iris/bitstream/handle/10665/92455/9789241506090_eng.pdf;jsessionid=0D27FD8BD63E539A0253273318D4CD4D?sequence=1

Wink, M. (2013). Evolution of secondary metabolites in legumes (Fabaceae). South African Journal of Botany, 89, 164-175. https://doi.org/10.1016/j.sajb.2013.06.006

Wynbrandt, J. (2000). The Excruciating History of Dentistry: Toothsome Tales and Oral Oddities from Babylon to Braces. New York: St. Martin's Griffin.

Chapter 2: The Discovery of Diethyl Ether as an Anaesthetic

al., T. K. (2009, November 8). Balloon rupture during coronary angioplasty causing dissection and intramural hematoma of the coronary artery; a case report. doi:10.1016/j.jccase.2009.06.002

Beringer, R. (2008, June). The Glostavent: Evolution of an Anaesthetic Machine for Developing Countries. Anaesthesia and Intensive Care , 36(3), 442-8. Retrieved May 6, 2021, from Richard Beringer.

Bhandari, S., Bhargava, A., Sharma, S., Keshwani, P., Sharma, R., & Banerjee, S. (2020, May 1). Clinical Profile of Covid-19 Infected Patients Admitted in a Tertiary Care Hospital in North India. 68(5), 13-17. Retrieved May 6, 2021, from https://europepmc.org/article/med/32610859

Encyclopedia.com. (2016, August). Cordus, Valerius. Retrieved May 6, 2021, from Encyclopedia: https://www.encyclopedia.com/people/science-and-technology/botany-biographies/valerius-cordus

Frercihs, R. R. (n.d.). Anesthesia and Queen Victoria. Retrieved May 5, 2021, from https://www.ph.ucla.edu/epi/snow/victoria.html

Haridas, R. P. (2013, November). Horace Wells' Demonstration of Nitrous Oxide in Boston . Anesthesiology, 119, 1014–1022. Retrieved May 5, 2021

McGill. (n.d.). Before ether was a potent painkiller, it was a hit with revellers. Retrieved May 6, 2021, from McGill: https://www.mcgill.ca/oss/article/drugs-health-news/ether-was-potent-painkiller-it-was-hit-revellers#:~:text=It%20was%20on%20Oct.,an%20inhaler%20he%20had%20devised.

Minkowski, W. L. (1992, February). Women healers of the middle ages: selected aspects of their history. American Journal of Public Health, 82(2), 288–295. doi:10.2105/ajph.82.2.288

O. Akenroye, O. O., Adebona, O. T., & Akenroye, A. T. (2013, December 3). Surgical Care in the Developing World-Strategies and Framework for Improvement. Journal of Public Health Africa, 4(2). Retrieved May 6, 2021, from https://www.ncbi.nlm.nih.gov/pmc/articles/PMC5345438/

Rössler, B., Marhofer, P., Hüpfl, M., Peterhans, B., & Schebesta, K. (2013, May). Preparedness of Anesthesiologists Working in Humanitarian Disasters. Disaster Medicine and Public Health Preparedness, 7(4), 408-412. Retrieved May 5, 2021

Science Direct. (1920, October). The effect of salt ingestion on cerebro-spinal fluid pressure and brain volume. American Journal of Physiology, 53(3), 464-476. doi:https://doi.org/10.1152/ajplegacy.1920.53.3.464

The Editors of Encyclopaedia Britannica. (1998, July 20). William Thomas Green Morton. Retrieved May 5, 2021, from

Encyclopaedia Britannica: https://www.britannica.com/biography/William-Thomas-Green-Morton

Watson, J., & Stetka, B. S. (2016, June 2). Opium to the OR: A Visual History of Anesthesia. Retrieved May 5, 2021, from Medscape: https://www.medscape.com/features/slideshow/history-of-anesthesia

Wood Library Museum. (n.d.). Schimmelbusch Mask. Retrieved May 5, 2021, from Wood Library Museum: https://www.woodlibrarymuseum.org/museum/schimmelbusch-mask/

Chapter 3: Everyday Use in Surgeries

Dallas, M. (2019). 8 Surprising Facts about Anesthesia. 87, 90-92 https://www.everydayhealth.com/news/surprising-facts-about-anesthesia/

Harrah, S. (2015). Medical Milestones: Discovery of Anesthesia & Timeline https://www.umhs-sk.org/blog/medical-milestones-discovery-anesthesia-timeline

Jakobsson, J. (2012). Anaesthesia for day case surgery. Oxford: Oxford University Press.

Mashour, G. A. (2009). Consciousness and awareness in anesthesia. Cambridge: Cambridge University Press.

Wilson, D. (2018). Advantages and Disadvantages of Anesthesia, 97, 125-130. https://emedicine.medscape.com/article/1271543-overview

Chapter 4: Local, Regional, and General Anesthesia

ASA. (2021). General Anesthesia: Definition & Side Effects - Made for This Moment. Made For This Moment | Anesthesia, Pain Management & Surgery. https://www.asahq.org/madeforthismoment/anesthesia-101/types-of-anesthesia/general-anesthesia/.

ASA. (2021). Local Anesthesia: Definition & Effects - Made for This Moment. Made For This Moment | Anesthesia, Pain Management & Surgery. https://www.asahq.org/

madeforthismoment/anesthesia-101/types-of-anesthesia/local-anesthesia/.

ASA. (2021). Regional Anesthesia: Definition & Effects - Made for This Moment. Made For This Moment | Anesthesia, Pain Management & Surgery. https://www.asahq.org/madeforthismoment/anesthesia-101/types-of-anesthesia/regional-anesthesia/.

ASA. (2021). Types of Anesthesia - Made for This Moment. Made For This Moment | Anesthesia, Pain Management & Surgery. https://www.asahq.org/madeforthismoment/anesthesia-101/types-of-anesthesia/.

Cleveland Clinic. (2020). Anesthesia: Anesthesiology, Surgery, Side Effects, Types, Risk. Cleveland Clinic. https://my.clevelandclinic.org/health/treatments/15286-anesthesia.

Guilding, C. (2019). Pharmacology Education Project. Anaesthetic drugs | Pharmacology Education Project. https://www.pharmacologyeducation.org/drugs/anaesthetic-drugs.

John Hopkins Medicine. (2021). Anesthesia. Johns Hopkins Medicine. https://www.hopkinsmedicine.org/health/treatment-tests-and-therapies/types-of-anesthesia-and-your-anesthesiologist.

Mayo Clinic. (2020). General anesthesia. Mayo Clinic. https://www.mayoclinic.org/tests-procedures/anesthesia/about/pac-20384568.

Trevor, A. J., Katzung, B. G., & Kruidering-Hall, M. (2015). In Katzung & Trevor's Pharmacology: Examination & Board Review, 11e (Vol. 11, pp. Part V-Chapter 25). essay, McGraw-Hill. https://accesspharmacy.mhmedical.com/Content.aspx?bookId=1568§ionId=95702505.

UCLA Health. (n.d.). Types of Anesthesia. UCLA Anesthesiology & Perioperative Medicine. https://www.uclahealth.org/anes/types-of-anesthesia#:~:text=There%20are%20four%20main%20categories,of%20anesthesia%20will%20be%20used.

Weatherspoon, D. (2018). General anesthesia: Side effects, risks, and stages. Medical News Today. https://www.medicalnewstoday.com/articles/265592#stages.

Whitlock, J., & Dhingra, J. A. (2020). Types of Anesthesia Used During Surgery. Verywell Health. https://www.verywellhealth.com/anesthesia-and-surgery-3157215.

Chapter 5: Common Anesthetics Today

Ferreira, A. L., Nunes, C., Mendes, J. G., & Amorim, P. (2019). Do we have today a reliable

method to detect the moment of loss of consciousness during induction of general anaesthesia? Revista Española de Anestesiología y Reanimación (English Edition), 66(2), 93–103.

Gadani, H., & Vyas, A. (2011). Anesthetic gases and global warming: Potentials, prevention and future of anesthesia. Department of Anesthesiology, M.P. Shah Medical College,, 5(1), 5-10. https://doi.org/10.4103/0259-1162.84171

Leake, C. (1925). The Historical Development of Surgical Anesthesia. The Scientific Monthly,

20(3), 304-328. Retrieved May 7, 2021, from http://www.jstor.org/stable/7173

Park, Y., & Kim, T. (n.d.). Anesthesia safety standards for operating rooms of small hospitals

and surgery clinics. J Korean Med Assoc, 63(9), 514-517. doi:https://doi.org/10.5124/jkma.2020.63.9.514

Chapter 6: Interactions with the Nervous System

Alberts, B. (1970, January 1). Ion Channels and the Electrical Properties of Membranes. Molecular Biology of the Cell. 4th edition. https://www.ncbi.nlm.nih.gov/books/NBK26910/.

Alkire, M. T., & Miller, J. (2005). General anesthesia and the neural correlates of consciousness. Progress in Brain Research, 229–597. https://doi.org/10.1016/s0079-6123(05)50017-7

Avila, A., Nguyen, L., & Rigo, J.-M. (2013). Glycine receptors and brain development. Frontiers in Cellular Neuroscience, 7. https://doi.org/10.3389/fncel.2013.00184

Cherry, K. (2020, January 16). Structure and Function of the Central Nervous System. Verywell Mind. https://www.verywellmind.com/what-is-the-central-nervous-system-2794981.

Cherry, K. (2020, June 4). What You Should Know About the Peripheral Nervous System. Verywell Mind. https://www.verywellmind.com/what-is-the-peripheral-nervous-system-2795465.

de Leon, A. S., & Tadi, P. (2020, July 10). Biochemistry, Gamma Aminobutyric Acid. StatPearls [Internet]. https://www.ncbi.nlm.nih.gov/books/NBK551683/#:~:text=%5B1%5D%20As%20an%20inhibitory%20neurotransmitter,excitatory%20postsynaptic%20potential%20(EPSP).

Lodish, H. (1970, January 1). Overview of Neuron Structure and Function. Molecular Cell Biology. 4th edition. https://www.ncbi.nlm.nih.gov/books/NBK21535/.

Mihic, S. J., Ye, Q., Wick, M. J., Koltchine, V. V., Krasowski, M. D., Finn, S. E., ... Harrison, N. L. (1997). Sites of alcohol and volatile anaesthetic action on GABAA and glycine receptors. Nature, 389(6649), 385–389. https://doi.org/10.1038/38738

Skaggs, W. E. (2013). Nervous system. Scholarpedia. http://www.scholarpedia.org/article/Nervous_system.

Son, Y. (2010). Molecular mechanisms of general anesthesia. Korean Journal of Anesthesiology, 59(1), 3. https://doi.org/10.4097/kjae.2010.59.1.3

Chapter 7: Anesthesia Awareness

American Society of Anesthesiologists. (2006). Practice Advisory for Intraoperative Awareness and Brain Function Monitoring: A Report by the American Society of Anesthesiologists Task Force on Intraoperative Awareness. Anesthesiology, 104(4), 847–864. https://doi.org/10.1097/00000542-200604000-00031

Bruchas, R. R., Kent, C. D., Wilson, H. D., & Domino, K. B. (2011). Anesthesia Awareness: Narrative Review of Psychological Sequelae, Treatment, and Incidence. Journal of Clinical Psychology in Medical Settings, 18(3), 257–267. https://doi.org/10.1007/s10880-011-9233-8

Chung, H. S. (2014). Awareness and recall during general anesthesia. Korean Journal of Anesthesiology, 66(5), 339–345. https://doi.org/10.4097/kjae.2014.66.5.339

Cook, T. M., Andrade, J., Bogod, D. G., Hitchman, J. M., Jonker, W. R., Lucas, N., Mackay, J. H., Nimmo, A. F., O'Connor, K., O'Sullivan, E. P., Paul, R. G., Palmer, J. H. M. G., Plaat, F., Radcliffe, J. J., Sury, M. R. J., Torevell, H. E., Wang, M., Hainsworth, J., Pandit, J. J., … on behalf of the Royal College of Anaesthetists and the Association of Anaesthetists of Great Britain and Ireland. (2014). 5th National Audit Project (NAP5) on accidental awareness during general anaesthesia: Patient experiences, human factors, sedation, consent, and medicolegal issues. BJA: British Journal of Anaesthesia, 113(4), 560–574. https://doi.org/10.1093/bja/aeu314

Eseonu, C. I., ReFaey, K., Garcia, O., John, A., Quiñones-Hinojosa, A., & Tripathi, P. (2017). Awake Craniotomy Anesthesia: A Comparison of the Monitored Anesthesia Care and Asleep-Awake-Asleep Techniques. World Neurosurgery, 104, 679–686. https://doi.org/10.1016/j.wneu.2017.05.053

Galley, H., & Hall, B. (2008). Films, facts and fiction. Anaesthesia, 63(7), 692–694. https://doi.org/10.1111/j.1365-2044.2008.05586.x

Garavaglia, M. M., Das, S., Cusimano, M. D., Crescini, C., Mazer, C. D., Hare, G. M. T., & Rigamonti, A. (2014). Anesthetic Approach to High-Risk Patients and Prolonged Awake Craniotomy Using Dexmedetomidine and Scalp Block. Journal of Neurosurgical Anesthesiology, 26(3), 226–233. https://doi.org/10.1097/ANA.0b013e3182a58aba

Harold, J. (Director). (2007). Awake [Film]. The Weinstein Company.

Kent, C. D., Mashour, G. A., Metzger, N. A., Posner, K. L., & Domino, K. B. (2013). Psychological impact of unexpected explicit recall of events occurring during surgery performed under sedation, regional anaesthesia, and general anaesthesia: Data from the Anesthesia Awareness Registry. British Journal of Anaesthesia, 110(3), 381–387. https://doi.org/10.1093/bja/aes386

Leslie, K., & Davidson, A. J. (2010). Awareness during anesthesia: A problem without solutions? Minerva Anestesiologica, 76(8), 624–628.

Martino, J., Honma, S. M., Findlay, A. M., Guggisberg, A. G., Kirsch, H. E., Berger, M. S., & Nagarajan, S. S. (2011). Resting functional connectivity in patients with brain tumors in eloquent areas. Annals of Neurology, 69(3), 521–532. https://doi.org/10.1002/ana.22167

Mashour, G. A., Wang, L. Y.-J., Turner, C. R., Vandervest, J. C., Shanks, A., & Tremper, K. K. (2009). A Retrospective Study of Intraoperative Awareness with Methodological Implications. Anesthesia & Analgesia, 108(2), 521–526. https://doi.org/10.1213/ane.0b013e3181732b0c

McCleane, G. J., & Cooper, R. (1990). The nature of pre-operative anxiety. Anaesthesia, 45(2), 153–155. https://doi.org/10.1111/j.1365-2044.1990.tb14285.x

Myles, P. S., Leslie, K., McNeil, J., Forbes, A., & Chan, M. T. V. (2004). Bispectral index monitoring to prevent awareness during anaesthesia: The B-Aware randomised controlled trial. The Lancet, 363(9423), 1757–1763. https://doi.org/10.1016/S0140-6736(04)16300-9

Orser, B. A., Mazer, C. D., & Baker, A. J. (2008). Awareness during anesthesia. CMAJ, 178(2), 185–188. https://doi.org/10.1503/cmaj.071761

Pandit, J. J., Andrade, J., Bogod, D. G., Hitchman, J. M., Jonker, W. R., Lucas, N., Mackay, J. H., Nimmo, A. F., O'Connor, K., O'Sullivan, E. P., Paul, R. G., Palmer, J. H. M. G., Plaat, F., Radcliffe, J. J., Sury, M. R. J., Torevell, H. E., Wang, M., Hainsworth, J., Cook, T. M., ... Association of Anaesthetists of Great Britain and Ireland. (2014). 5th National Audit Project (NAP5) on accidental awareness during general anaesthesia: Summary of main findings and risk factors. British Journal of Anaesthesia, 113(4), 549–559. https://doi.org/10.1093/bja/aeu313

Pandit, J. J., Russell, I. F., & Wang, M. (2015). Interpretations of responses using the isolated forearm technique in general anaesthesia: A debate. BJA: British Journal of Anaesthesia, 115(suppl_1), i32–i45. https://doi.org/10.1093/bja/aev106

Piai, V., Vos, S. H., Idelberger, R., Gans, P., Doorduin, J., & Ter Laan, M. (2019). Awake Surgery for a Violin Player: Monitoring Motor and Music Performance, A Case Report. Archives of Clinical Neuropsychology: The Official Journal of the National Academy of Neuropsychologists, 34(1), 132–137. https://doi.org/10.1093/arclin/acy009

Piccioni, F., & Fanzio, M. (2008). Management of anesthesia in awake craniotomy. Minerva Anestesiologica, 74(7-8), 393–408.

Reuters, T. (2020, February 19). Violinist plays Mahler and Gershwin as surgeons remove brain tumour. CBC. https://www.cbc.ca/news/health/violinist-brain-surgery-1.5468467

Samuelsson, P., Brudin, L., & Sandin, R. H. (2007). Late psychological symptoms after awareness among consecutively included surgical patients. Anesthesiology, 106(1), 26–32. https://doi.org/10.1097/00000542-200701000-00009

Sandin, R. H., Enlund, G., Samuelsson, P., & Lennmarken, C. (2000). Awareness during anaesthesia: A prospective case study. The Lancet, 355(9205), 707–711. https://doi.org/10.1016/S0140-6736(99)11010-9

Sebel, P. S., Bowdle, T. A., Ghoneim, M. M., Rampil, I. J., Padilla, R. E., Gan, T. J., & Domino, K. B. (2004). The incidence of awareness during anesthesia: A multicenter United States study. Anesthesia and Analgesia, 99(3), 833–839, table of contents. https://doi.org/10.1213/01.ANE.0000130261.90896.6C

Sury, M. R. J. (2016). Accidental awareness during anesthesia in children. Pediatric Anesthesia, 26(5), 468–474. https://doi.org/10.1111/pan.12894

Tasbihgou, S. R., Vogels, M. F., & Absalom, A. R. (2018). Accidental awareness during general anaesthesia – a narrative review. Anaesthesia, 73(1), 112–122. https://doi.org/10.1111/anae.14124

Wang, M., Messina, A. G., & Russell, I. F. (2012). The topography of awareness: A classification of intra-operative cognitive states. Anaesthesia, 67(11), 1197–1201. https://doi.org/10.1111/anae.12041

Chapter 8: Can Hypnosis Replace Anesthesia?

Bruno, D. (2019). Hypnotherapy isn't magic, but it helps some patients cope with surgery and recovery. The Washington Post. Retrieved 6 May 2021, from https://www.washingtonpost.com/health/hypnotherapy-as-an-alternative-to-anesthesia-some-patients--and-doctors--say-yes/2019/11/08/046bc1d2-e53f-11e9-b403-f738899982d2_story.html.

Cozzolino, M., Celia, G., Rossi, K., & Rossi, E. (2020). Hypnosis as Sole Anesthesia for Dental Removal in a Patient with Multiple Chemical Sensitivity. International Journal of Clinical and Experimental Hypnosis, 68(3), 371–383. https://doi.org/10.1080/00207144.2020.1762494

Drouet, N., & Chedeau, G. (2016). Hypnopraxia, a new hypnotic technique for hypnoanesthesia. Journal of Clinical Anesthesia, 37, 14–16. https://doi.org/10.1016/j.jclinane.2016.10.039

Holden, A. (2012). The art of suggestion: the use of hypnosis in dentistry. British Dental Journal, 212(11), 549–551. https://doi.org/10.1038/sj.bdj.2012.467

Ketterhagen, D., VandeVusse, L., & Berner, M. (2002). Self-Hypnosis: Alternative Anesthesia for Childbirth. MCN, the American Journal of Maternal Child Nursing, 27(6), 335–340. https://doi.org/10.1097/00005721-200211000-00007

Kuttner, L. (2012). Pediatric hypnosis: pre-, peri-, and post-anesthesia: Pediatric hypnosis. Pediatric Anesthesia, 22(6), 573–577. https://doi.org/10.1111/j.1460-9592.2012.03860.x

Lacroix, C., Duhoux, F., Bettendorff, J., Watremez, C., Roelants, F., Docquier, M., Potié, A., Coyette, M., Gerday, A., Samartzi, V., Piette, P., Piette, N., & Berliere, M. (2019). Impact of Perioperative Hypnosedation on Postmastectomy Chronic Pain: Preliminary Results. Integrative Cancer Therapies, 18,

1534735419869494–1534735419869494. https://doi.org/
10.1177/1534735419869494

Lankton, S. (2016). Conscious/Unconscious Dissociation
Induction: Increasing Hypnotic Performance With "Resistant"
Clients. The American Journal of Clinical Hypnosis, 59(2),
175–185. https://doi.org/10.1080/00029157.2017.1210408

Lankton, S. (2020). What Milton Erickson said about being
Ericksonian. The American Journal of Clinical Hypnosis,
63(1), 4–13. https://doi.org/10.1080/00029157.2020.1754068

Maquet, P., Faymonville, M., Degueldre, C., Delfiore, G.,
Franck, G., Luxen, A., & Lamy, M. (1999). Functional
neuroanatomy of hypnotic state. Biological Psychiatry (1969),
45(3), 327–333. https://doi.org/10.1016/S0006-
3223(97)00546-5

Manyande, A., Cyna, A., Yip, P., Chooi, C., Middleton, P., &
Cyna, A. (2015). Non-pharmacological interventions for
assisting the induction of anaesthesia in children. Cochrane
Library, 2015(7), CD006447–CD006447. https://doi.org/
10.1002/14651858.CD006447.pub3

Stone, A., Sheinberg, R., Bertram, A., & Seymour, A. (2016).
Are Anesthesia Providers Ready for Hypnosis? Anesthesia
Providers' Attitudes Toward Hypnotherapy. The American
Journal of Clinical Hypnosis, 58(4), 411–418. https://doi.org/
10.1080/00029157.2015.1136589

Vanhaudenhuyse, A., Laureys, S., & Faymonville, M. (2013).
Neurophysiology of hypnosis. Neurophysiologie Clinique,
44(4), 343–353. https://doi.org/10.1016/j.neucli.2013.09.006

Von Ungern-Sternberg, B., & Habre, W. (2009). Hypnosis as
an alternative to avoid general anesthesia in a child with
severe pulmonary arterial hypertension. Pediatric Anesthesia,
19(2), 182–183. https://doi.org/10.1111/j.1460-
9592.2008.02800.x

Wobst, A. (2007). Hypnosis and surgery: Past, present, and
future. Anesthesia and Analgesia, 104(5), 1199–1208. https://
doi.org/10.1213/01.ane.0000260616.49050.6d

Wolf, T., Wolf, D., Callaway, A., Below, D., d'Hoedt, B., Willershausen, B., & Daubländer, M. (2016). Hypnosis and Local Anesthesia for Dental Pain Relief-Alternative or Adjunct Therapy?-A Randomized, Clinical-Experimental Crossover Study. International Journal of Clinical and Experimental Hypnosis, 64(4), 391–403. https://doi.org/10.1080/00207144.2016.1209033

Chapter 9: Narcotics as Anesthetics

Agenas I, Gustafsson L, Rane A, Sawe J. (1982). Analgetikaterapi for cancerpatienter. Lakartidningen, 79, 287–289

Afsharimani, B., Cabot, P., & Parat, M.-O. (2011). Morphine and tumor growth and metastasis. Cancer and Metastasis Reviews, 30(2), 225–238. https://doi.org/10.1007/s10555-011-9285-0

Bandyopadhyay S. (2019). An 8,000-year history of use and abuse of opium and opioids: how that matters for a successful control of the epidemic? Neurology,9 (Suppl. 15), 9 -55.

Brohan, J., & Goudra, B. G. (2017). The Role of GABA Receptor Agonists in Anesthesia and Sedation. CNS Drugs, 31(10), 845–856. https://doi.org/10.1007/s40263-017-0463-7

Brownstein, M. J. (1993). A brief history of opiates, opioid peptides, and opioid receptors. Proceedings of the National Academy of Sciences, 90(12), 5391–5393. https://doi.org/10.1073/pnas.90.12.5391

Eddy, N. B. (1957). The History of the Development of Narcotics. Law and Contemporary Problems, 22(1), 3. https://doi.org/10.2307/1190429

Egan, T. D. (2019). Are opioids indispensable for general anaesthesia? British Journal of Anaesthesia, 122(6). https://doi.org/10.1016/j.bja.2019.02.018

Egan, T. D., & Svensen, C. H. (2018). Multimodal General Anesthesia. Anesthesia & Analgesia, 127(5), 1104–1106. https://doi.org/10.1213/ane.0000000000003743

Ferry N, Dhanjal S. (2021). Opioid Anesthesia. StatPearls Publishing. https://www.ncbi.nlm.nih.gov/books/NBK532956/

Forget, P. (2019). Opioid-free anaesthesia. Why and how? A contextual analysis. Anaesthesia Critical Care & Pain Medicine, 38(2), 169–172. https://doi.org/10.1016/j.accpm.2018.05.002

History.com Editors. (2017, June 12). Heroin, Morphine and Opiates. History.com. https://www.history.com/topics/crime/history-of-heroin-morphine-and-opiates.

Kritikos, P. G., & Papadaki, S. P. (1967, January 1). UNODC - Bulletin on Narcotics - 1967 Issue 3 - 003. United Nations : Office on Drugs and Crime. https://www.unodc.org/unodc/en/data-and-analysis/bulletin/bulletin_1967-01-01_3_page004.html.

Lu, L., Fang, Y., & Wang, X. (2007). Drug Abuse in China: Past, Present and Future. Cellular and Molecular Neurobiology, 28(4), 479–490. https://doi.org/10.1007/s10571-007-9225-2

Nakhaee, S., Ghasemi, S., Karimzadeh, K., Zamani, N., Alinejad-Mofrad, S., & Mehrpour, O. (2020). The effects of opium on the cardiovascular system: a review of side effects, uses, and potential mechanisms. Substance Abuse Treatment, Prevention, and Policy, 15(1). https://doi.org/10.1186/s13011-020-00272-8

Nambiar, N. (2020, November 26). Analgesia vs. Anesthesia: Learn the Differences. eMediHealth. https://www.emedihealth.com/analgesia-vs-anesthesia.html.

Netherland, J., & Hansen, H. B. (2016). The War on Drugs That Wasn't: Wasted Whiteness, "Dirty Doctors," and Race in Media Coverage of Prescription Opioid Misuse. Culture, Medicine, and Psychiatry, 40(4), 664–686. https://doi.org/10.1007/s11013-016-9496-5

Opium: Uses, Addiction Treatment & Side Effects. Drugs.com. (n.d.). https://www.drugs.com/illicit/opium.html.

Rojas-Pérez-Ezquerra, P., Micozzi, S., Torrado-Español, I., Rodríguez-Fernández, A., Albéndiz-Gutiérrez, V., &

Noguerado-Mellado, B. (2019). Allergic Contact Dermatitis to Fentanyl TTS with Good Tolerance to Systemic Fentanyl. Recent Patents on Inflammation & Allergy Drug Discovery, 13(1), 66–68. https://doi.org/10.2174/1872213x13666190527105718

Rosenblum, A., Marsch, L. A., Joseph, H., & Portenoy, R. K. (2008). Opioids and the treatment of chronic pain: Controversies, current status, and future directions. Experimental and Clinical Psychopharmacology, 16(5), 405–416. https://doi.org/10.1037/a0013628

Roy, S., Wang, J., Kelschenbach, J., Koodie, L., & Martin, J. (2006). Modulation of Immune Function by Morphine: Implications for Susceptibility to Infection. Journal of Neuroimmune Pharmacology, 1(1), 77–89. https://doi.org/10.1007/s11481-005-9009-8

Russell, N. J. W., Schaible, H.-G., & Schmidt, R. F. (1987). Opiates inhibit the discharges of fine afferent units from inflamed knee joint of the cat. Neuroscience Letters, 76(1), 107–112. https://doi.org/10.1016/0304-3940(87)90201-1

Sacerdote, P., Bianchi, M., Gaspani, L., Manfredi, B., Maucione, A., Terno, G., ... Panerai, A. E. (2000). The Effects of Tramadol and Morphine on Immune Responses and Pain After Surgery in Cancer Patients. Anesthesia & Analgesia, 90(6), 1411–1414. https://doi.org/10.1097/00000539-200006000-00028

Schiff, Paul. (2001). Opium and Its Alkaloids. American Journal of Pharmaceutical Education. 66.

Schwenk, E. S., & Mariano, E. R. (2018). Designing the ideal perioperative pain management plan starts with multimodal analgesia. Korean Journal of Anesthesiology, 71(5), 345–352. https://doi.org/10.4097/kja.d.18.00217

Vella-Brincat, J., & MacLeod, A. D. (2007). Adverse Effects of Opioids on the Central Nervous Systems of Palliative Care Patients. Journal of Pain & Palliative Care Pharmacotherapy, 21(1), 15–25. https://doi.org/10.1080/j354v21n01_05